Neonatal Nursing: Clinical Concepts and Practice Implications, Part 1

Editor

LESLIE ALTIMIER

CRITICAL CARE NURSING CLINICS OF NORTH AMERICA

www.ccnursing.theclinics.com

March 2024 • Volume 36 • Number 1

ELSEVIER

1600 John F. Kennedy Boulevard • Suite 1800 • Philadelphia, Pennsylvania, 19103-2899

http://www.theclinics.com

CRITICAL CARE NURSING CLINICS OF NORTH AMERICA Volume 36, Number 1
March 2024 ISSN 0899-5885, ISBN-13: 978-0-443-13121-9

Editor: Kerry Holland
Developmental Editor: Shivank Joshi

Critical Care Nursing Clinics of North America (ISSN 0899-5885) is published quarterly by Elsevier Inc., 360 Park Avenue South, New York, NY 10010-1710. Months of issue are March, June, September, and December. Business and Editorial Offices: 1600 John F. Kennedy Blvd., Suite 1800, Philadelphia, PA 19103-2899. Periodicals postage paid at New York, NY and additional mailing offices. Subscription prices are $166.00 per year for US individuals, $100.00 per year for US students and residents, $206.00 per year for Canadian individuals, $230.00 per year for international individuals, $115.00 per year for international students/residents and $100.00 per year for Canadian students/residents. For institutional access pricing please contact Customer Service via the contact information below. To receive student/resident rate, orders must be accompanied by name of affiliated institution, data of term, and the *signature* of program/residency coordinator on institution letterhead. Orders will be billed at individual rate until proof of status is received. Foreign air speed delivery is included in all *Clinics* subscription prices. All prices are subject to change without notice. **POSTMASTER:** Send address changes to *Critical Care Nursing Clinics of North America*, Elsevier Health Sciences Division, Subscription Customer Service, 3251 Riverport Lane, Maryland Heights, MO 63043. **Customer Service: 1-800-654-2452 (US and Canada); 314-447-8871 (outside US and Canada). Fax: 314-447-8029. E-mail:** JournalsCustomerService-usa@elsevier.com **(for print support) and** JournalsOnlineSupport-usa@elsevier.com **(for online support).**

Reprints. For copies of 100 or more of articles in this publication, please contact the Commercial Reprints Department, Elsevier Inc., 360 Park Avenue South, New York, New York, 10010-1710; Tel.: 212-633-3874, Fax: 212-633-3820, and E-mail: reprints@elsevier.com.

Critical Care Nursing Clinics of North America is covered in *MEDLINE/PubMed (Index Medicus), International Nursing Index, Nursing Citation Index, Cumulative Index to Nursing and Allied Health Literature, and RNdex Top 100.*

Contributors

EDITOR

LESLIE ALTIMIER, DNP, RN, NE-BC, MSN, BSN
Regional Director of Neonatal Services, Cardinal Glennon Children's Hospital, St Louis, Missouri, USA

AUTHORS

LESLIE ALTIMIER, DNP, RN, NE-BC, MSN, BSN
Regional Director of Neonatal Services, Cardinal Glennon Children's Hospital, St Louis, Missouri, USA

MARION BENDIXEN, PhD, MSN, RN, IBCLC
Professor, College of Nursing, University of Florida, Gainesville, Florida, USA

MANOJ BINIWALE, MBBS, MD
Division of Neonatology, Department of Pediatrics, Keck School of Medicine of USC, Los Angeles General Medical Center, Los Angeles, California, USA

MARINA BOYKOVA, PhD, RN, PNAP
Board Member, Council of International Neonatal Nurses, Inc (COINN), Associate Professor, School of Nursing and Health Sciences, Holy Family University, Philadelphia, Pennsylvania, USA

HUSSAH BUBSHAIT, RN, MSN
Professor, College of Nursing, University of Florida, Gainesville, Florida, USA

TARAH T. COLAIZY, MD, MPH
Division of Neonatology, Department of Pediatrics, The University of Iowa, University of Iowa Stead Family Children's Hospital, Iowa City, Iowa, USA

JOHN M. DAGLE, MD, PhD
Division of Neonatology, Department of Pediatrics, The University of Iowa, University of Iowa Stead Family Children's Hospital, Iowa City, Iowa, USA

STEPHANIE DIGGS, MD
Division of Newborn Medicine, Department of Pediatrics, Washington University School of Medicine, St Louis, Missouri, USA

ANDREW K. EWER, MD, MRCP, FRCPCH
Professor, Institute of Metabolism and Systems Research, College of Medical and Dental Sciences, University of Birmingham, Birmingham, United Kingdom

ALISSANDRE EUGENE, BS
Professor, College of Nursing, University of Florida, Gainesville, Florida, USA

KELIY FORDHAM RN, BSN
Professor, College of Nursing, University of Florida, Gainesville, Florida, USA

KELLI GARBER, DNP, APRN, PPCNP-BC
Clinical Assistant Professor, Director of DNP Advanced Practice Program, Old Dominion University School of Nursing, Virginia Beach, Virginia, USA

ADRIENNE GEFRE
Professor, College of Nursing, University of Florida, Gainesville, Florida, USA

ANURAG GIRDHAR, DCh, DNB, MRCPCH
Department of Neonatology, Birmingham Women's Hospital NHS Trust, Birmingham, United Kingdom

HEIDI M. HARMON, MD
Division of Neonatology, Department of Pediatrics, The University of Iowa, University of Iowa Stead Family Children's Hospital, Iowa City, Iowa, USA

MELODY HERNANDEZ, MD, PhD, RN
NICU Nurse Telehealth Scientist, Nicklaus Children's Hospital, Miami, Florida, USA

STEPHEN K. HUNTER, MD, PhD
Department of Obstetrics and Gynecology, The University of Iowa, Iowa City, Iowa, USA

CAROLE KENNER, PhD, RN, FAAN, FNAP, ANEF, IDFCOINN
Chief Executive Officer, Council of International Neonatal Nurses, Inc (COINN), Dean, School of Nursing and Health Sciences, The College of New Jersey, Ewing, New Jersey, USA

JONATHAN M. KLEIN, MD
Division of Neonatology, Department of Pediatrics, The University of Iowa, University of Iowa Stead Family Children's Hospital, Iowa City, Iowa, USA

REBECCA KOERNER, PhD, APRN, CPNP-PC
Professor, College of Nursing, University of Florida, Gainesville, Florida, USA

TERRI MARIN, PhD, NNP-BC, FAAN, FANNP, FNAP
Associate Professor, Department of Nursing Science, Augusta University College of Nursing, Augusta, Georgia, USA

YUI MATSUDA, PhD, PHNA-BC, MPH
Associate Professor of Clinical, University of Miami School of Nursing and Health Studies, Coral Gables, Florida, USA

ERIN J. MAYS, MSN, APRN, NNP-BC
St. Louis Children's Hospital NICU, St Louis, Missouri, USA

STEVE J. McELROY, MD
Division of Neonatology, Department of Pediatrics, University of California, Davis, Sacramento, California, USA

PATRICK J. McNAMARA, MD, MSc
Division of Neonatology, Departments of Pediatrics and Internal Medicine, The University of Iowa, University of Iowa Stead Family Children's Hospital, Iowa City, Iowa, USA

JAMES MOORE, MD, PhD
Department of Pediatrics, Division of Neonatology, University of Connecticut School of Medicine, Hartford, Connecticut, USA

CRISTIAN EMANUEL MUÑOZ, RN
Instructor of Neonatology, Iberoamerican Society of Neonatology (SIBEN), Belgrano, San Luis, Argentina

LESLIE A. PARKER, PhD, APRN
Professor, College of Nursing, University of Florida, Gainesville, Florida, USA

RANGASAMY RAMANATHAN, MBBS, DCH, MD
Professor of Pediatrics, Chief, Division of Neonatology, Department of Pediatrics, Keck School of Medicine of USC, Los Angeles General Medical Center, Los Angeles, California, USA

DANIELLE ALTARES SARIK, PhD, APRN, CPNP-PC
Director of Nursing Research and Evidence-Based Practice, Nicklaus Children's Hospital, Miami, Florida, USA

AUGUSTO SOLA, MD
Professor of Neonatology, Iberoamerican Society of Neonatology (SIBEN), Wellington, Florida, USA

DEBORAH STEWARD, PhD, RN
Associate Professor Emeritus, The Ohio State University College of Nursing, Columbus, Ohio, USA

STEPHANIE SYKES, DNP, APRN-CNP, NNP-BC
Assistant Clinical Professor, Director, Neonatal Nurse Practitioner Specialty Track, The Ohio State University College of Nursing, Columbus, Ohio, USA

MARÍA TERESA MONTES BUENO, RN
Professor of Neonatology, Iberoamerican Society of Neonatology (SIBEN), Madrid, Spain

EVELYN ABRAHANTE TERRELL, OTD, MHSA
Director of Telehealth and Special Projects, Nicklaus Children's Hospital, Miami, Florida, USA

JODI ULLOA, DNP, APRN-CNP, NNP-BC
Assistant Clinical Professor, The Ohio State University College of Nursing, Columbus, Ohio, USA

ZACHARY A. VESOULIS, MD, MS
Division of Newborn Medicine, Department of Pediatrics, Washington University School of Medicine, St Louis, Missouri, USA

BARBARA WARNER, MD, MS
Division of Newborn Medicine, Department of Pediatrics, Washington University School of Medicine, St Louis, Missouri, USA

ROBERT D. WHITE, MD
Director, Regional Newborn Program, Beacon Children's Hospital, South Bend, Indiana, USA

CATHERINE LEWIS WITT, PhD, NNP-BC
Dean, Professor, Loretto Heights School of Nursing, Regis University, Denver, Colorado, USA

Contents

Preface: Neonatal Nursing: Clinical Concepts and Practice Implications   xiii

Leslie Altimier

Dangerous Things We Used to Do in Neonatology   1

Catherine Lewis Witt

Neonatology has been a rapidly growing specialty, starting in the early 1900s with premature infants displayed in incubator shows, to today with complex disease processes treated in state-of-the-art neonatal intensive care units. Along the way evolving knowledge, medications, and technology provided opportunities to learn from mistakes and misguided treatments. The ability to learn from past mistakes improves our care now and illustrates the need for humility and vigilance in everything we do. This article explores errors made in the past as we look forward to the future.

The Effects of Health Disparities on Neonatal Outcomes   11

Erin J. Mays, Stephanie Diggs, Zachary A. Vesoulis, and Barbara Warner

The history of racism in the United States was established with slavery, and the carry-over effect continues to impact health care through structural and institutional racism. Racial segregation and redlining have impacted access to quality health care, thereby impacting prematurity and infant mortality rates. Health disparities also impact neonatal morbidities such as intraventricular hemorrhage and necrotizing enterocolitis and the family care experience including the establishment of breastfeeding and health care provider interactions.

Care from Birth to Discharge of Infants Born at 22 to 23 Weeks' Gestation   23

John M. Dagle, Stephen K. Hunter, Tarah T. Colaizy, Steve J. McElroy, Heidi M. Harmon, Patrick J. McNamara, and Jonathan M. Klein

The clinical care of infants born at 22 weeks' gestation must be well-designed and standardized if optimal results are to be expected. Although several approaches to care in this vulnerable population are possible, protocols should be neither random nor inconsistent. We describe the approach taken at the University of Iowa Stead Family Children's Hospital neonatal intensive care unit with respect to preterm infants born at 22 weeks' gestation. We have chosen to present our standardize care plan with respect to prenatal, neurologic, nutritional, gastrointestinal, and skin management. Respiratory and cardiopulmonary care will be briefly reviewed, as these strategies have been published previously.

Couplet Care—The Next Frontier of Care in the Newborn Intensive Care Unit   35

Robert D. White

> Couplet care of mother and newborn intensive care unit (NICU) baby in the same room is a new, rapidly evolving option for the care of NICU babies. This change has structural and operational challenges that require careful planning but its successful implementation is likely to drive enhanced family participation in the care of their baby throughout the NICU stay as well as improve collaboration between obstetric and neonatal providers.

Understanding Near-Infrared Spectroscopy: An Update   41

Terri Marin and James Moore

> Near-infrared spectroscopy (NIRS) is a novel technology that uses infrared light to noninvasively and continuously measure regional oxygen extraction in real time at the bedside. Neonatal research using this device supports its use as an adjunct to routine cardiovascular monitoring because NIRS serves as a surrogate marker for end-organ perfusion and can detect minute changes in cerebral, intestinal, and kidney tissue beds. Multiple conditions affecting premature infants are frequently associated with hypoperfusion; therefore, methods to detect early tissue-specific perfusion alterations may substantially improve the clinician's ability to intervene and prevent further deterioration.

Noninvasive Ventilation   51

Rangasamy Ramanathan and Manoj Biniwale

> Systematic Reviews and Randomized clinical trials have shown that the use of noninvasive ventilation (NIV) compared to invasive mechanical ventilation reduces the risk of bronchopulmonary dysplasia and or mortality. Most commonly used NIV modes include nasal continuous positive airway pressure, bi-phasic modes, such as, bi-level positive airway pressure, nasal intermittent positive pressure ventilation, high flow nasal cannula, noninvasive neurally adjusted ventilatory assist, and nasal high frequency ventilation are discussed in this review.

Monitoring SpO$_2$: The Basics of Retinopathy of Prematurity (Back to Basics) and Targeting Oxygen Saturation   69

Augusto Sola, Leslie Altimier, María Teresa Montes Bueno, and Cristian Emanuel Muñoz

> Oxygen (O2) is a drug frequently used in newborn care. Adverse effects of hypoxia are well known but the damaging effects of excess oxygen administration and oxidative stress have only been studied in the last 2 decades. Many negative effects have been described, including retinopathy of prematurity . Noninvasive pulse oximetry (SpO2) is useful to detect hypoxemia but requires careful evaluation and understanding of the frequently changing relationship between O2 and hemoglobin to prevent hyperoxemia. Intention to treat SpO2 ranges should be individualized for every newborn receiving supplemental O2, according to gestational age, post-natal age, and clinical condition.

Pulse Oximetry Screening for Critical Congenital Heart Defects in Newborn Babies   99

Anurag Girdhar and Andrew K. Ewer

Pulse oximetry screening (POS) was first described over 20 years ago. However, in recent years, major clinical trials have demonstrated consistent test accuracy for the detection of critical congenital heart defects (CCHD). International uptake of POS has progressed well over the last 10 years with most major high-income countries now recommending screening. This review describes the evidence base which has led to this, the current debate regarding choice of screening algorithm, and the future areas for further research.

Midline Catheter Use in the Neonatal Intensive Care Unit   111

Stephanie Sykes, Jodi Ulloa, and Deborah Steward

Neonates admitted to the neonatal intensive care unit (NICU) are a unique population who most often begin life acutely or critically ill. Venous access is required by most acutely/critically ill neonates, especially those born preterm. Access is required for implementing management strategies such as stabilization, medications, fluids, nutrition, and transfusion of blood products. However, achieving and maintaining venous access in these neonates can be difficult, especially in preterm infants due to a myriad of contributing factors. Peripheral intravenous (PIV) catheters and peripherally inserted central catheters (PICC) are 2 common vascular access approaches used in the NICU and have traditionally been the most studied in the neonatal literature. Both options offer advantages and disadvantages. An alternative to PIVs and PICCs is the midline peripheral catheter (MPC), which in the literature may also be referred to as extended dwell peripheral intravenous catheters. Depending on the intended use, the MPC offers a venous access approach between a PIV and PICC. Usage of MPCs in the NICU is slowly increasing with the limited published evidence suggesting they are viable option when considering the need for vascular access. The purpose of this article is to present the advantages and disadvantages of MPCs as an alternative approach for venous access in neonates when appropriate.

Mother's Own Milk Versus Donor Human Milk: What's the Difference?   119

Leslie A. Parker, Rebecca Koernere, Keliy Fordham, Hussah Bubshait, Alissandre Eugene, Adrienne Gefre, and Marion Bendixen

Mother's own milk (MOM) is known to decrease complications in preterm infants and when unavailable, it is recommended that preterm very low–birth weight infants be fed donor human milk (DHM). Due to the pasteurization, processing, and lactation stage of donors, DHM does not contain the same nutritional, immunologic, and microbial components as MOM. This review summarizes the differences between MOM and DHM, the potential effects on health outcomes, and the clinical implications of these differences. Finally, implications for research and clinical practice are discussed.

Perspectives on Telehealth Use with the Neonatal Population: Policy, Practice, and Implementation Considerations   135

Danielle Altares Sarik, Yui Matsuda, Kelli Garber, Melody Hernandez, and Evelyn Abrahante Terrell

Telehealth has proven to be a valuable approach to providing care to the neonatal population, including supporting families during the transition to home, facilitating remote monitoring of fragile neonates, and connecting neonatal experts with infants and caregivers in underserved or remote communities. Clinicians engaging in telehealth need to be aware of policies and regulations that govern practice as well as the potential health equity issues that may present themselves.

Neonatal Nursing Care from a Global Perspective   **147**

Carole Kenner and Marina Boykova

Neonatal nurses play an essential role in small and sick newborn care. In the last few years, especially during the pandemic, neonatal mortality stayed relatively static. Recognition is growing that neonatal nurses represent a specialty that requires unique, consistent, competency-based training and education to provide the best possible care. The Council of International Neonatal Nurses, Inc collaborates with many global stakeholders to raise the standards of neonatal nursing care, especially in Africa.

CRITICAL CARE NURSING
CLINICS OF NORTH AMERICA

FORTHCOMING ISSUES

June 2024
**Neonatal Nursing: Clinical Concepts and
Practice Implications, Part 2**
Leslie Altimier, *Editor*

September 2024
**Moving Forward in Critical Care Nursing:
Lessons Learned from the COVID-19
Pandemic**
Sharon O'Donoghue and Justin DiLibero,
Editors

December 2024
Pain Management
Lynn C. Parsons, *Editor*

RECENT ISSUES

December 2023
Older Adults in Critical Care
Deborah Garbee, *Editor*

September 2023
Pediatric Intensive Care Nursing
Melissa Ferniz Nunn, *Editor*

June 2023
Evidenced-Based Trauma Pearls
Jeanette Vaughan and Whitney Villegas,
Editors

SERIES OF RELATED INTEREST

Nursing Clinics of North America http://www.nursing.theclinics.com

THE CLINICS ARE AVAILABLE ONLINE!
Access your subscription at:
www.theclinics.com

Preface

Neonatal Nursing: Clinical Concepts and Practice Implications

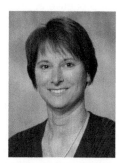

Leslie Altimier, DNP, RN, NE-BC, MSN, BSN
Editor

This issue, dedicated to neonates, is Part I of a two-part series providing a comprehensive overview of current and future changes in clinical practice. Most Neonatal Intensive Care Units (NICUs) now have cohesive multidisciplinary teams that function within a uniform unit culture. Nursing is an integral component of that team and has been at the forefront by embracing and integrating these changes. Investing in new and emerging technologies can support providers in optimizing care and could improve training, safety, and neonatal outcomes.

Care for preterm infants has improved considerably in the last decades, and although outcomes have improved, prematurity is still a large global health issue and is ranked in the top 10 of the World Health Organization's list of leading causes of burden of disease. In the early 1900s, premature infants were displayed in incubator shows. It is hard to believe that only a century ago, most premature infants were sent home from the hospital without any special interventions and many of these children did not survive past their first birthday. This issue of *Critical Care Nursing Clinics of North America* presents a further look at the dangerous things we used to do in Neonatology.

Great emphasis is now on Social Determinants of Health (SDOH), which have a major impact on people's health, well-being, and quality of life. SDOH are the conditions in the environments where people are born, live, learn, work, play, worship, and age that affect a wide range of health, functioning, and quality-of-life outcomes and risks. Disparities begin to impact children before they are born, at birth, and after birth. The first step in dismantling health disparities is acknowledging the presence of deeply

Crit Care Nurs Clin N Am 36 (2024) xiii–xvi
https://doi.org/10.1016/j.cnc.2023.11.009
0899-5885/24/© 2023 Published by Elsevier Inc.

ccnursing.theclinics.com

embedded racism and its long-standing impact on health care in minority populations, which is a topic of this issue. Much work has gone into studying the effects of health disparities on neonatal outcomes and is shared here in this issue focused on Neonatology.

Successful outcomes of extremely premature infants do not begin in the NICU, nor do they rely solely on neonatal interventions. The path to achieving outstanding outcomes begins before birth and involves collaboration and coordination of practices developed by maternal-fetal-medicine physicians with those developed by neonatologists. The clinical care of infants born at 22 weeks' gestation must be well-designed and standardized if optimal results are to be expected. A proactive approach must begin before birth and continue throughout the hospitalization to minimize variability in how the medical and nursing teams care for infants born below 24 weeks' gestation. Although several approaches to care for this vulnerable population are possible, protocols should be neither random nor inconsistent. A standardized care approach will describe neonatal care in regard to prenatal, neurologic, nutritional, gastrointestinal, and skin management. Respiratory and cardiopulmonary care is briefly reviewed.

Many changes have occurred since then. The NICU of the past was closed off and very restrictive. Over the years, there have been many changes, not only in technology but also in the environment in which we care for vulnerable babies and their families. Couplet care of mother and NICU baby in the same room is a new, rapidly evolving option for the care of NICU babies. This change has structural and operational challenges that require careful planning, but its successful implementation is likely to drive enhanced family participation in the care of their baby throughout the NICU stay as well as improve collaboration between obstetric and neonatal providers.

Technology has brought in new infant MRI machines for easy diagnosis and improving treatment plans. PET scans and radionucleate scanners like HIDA, DMSA, and DTPA help in tracking the overall health of the neonate without causing any physical pain. Continuous electroencephalography monitoring is being used to optimize neurodevelopment, as is near-infrared spectroscopy (NIRS) for cerebral and splanchnic blood flow monitoring.

NIRS is a novel technology discussed in this issue. NIRS uses infrared light to noninvasively and continuously measure regional oxygen (O_2) extraction in real-time at the bedside. Neonatal research using this device supports its use as an adjunct to routine cardiovascular monitoring, as NIRS serves as a surrogate marker for end-organ perfusion, and can detect minute changes in cerebral, intestinal, and kidney tissue beds. Multiple conditions affecting premature infants are frequently associated with hypoperfusion; therefore, methods to detect early tissue-specific perfusion alterations may substantially improve the clinician's ability to intervene and prevent further deterioration.

As technology advances, there has been more research in fine-tuning respiratory support and moving from highly technical invasive mechanical ventilation (IMV) to noninvasive ventilation (NIV), although methods of NIV have also become highly technical. Studies have demonstrated that the use of NIV compared with IMV reduces the risk of bronchopulmonary dysplasia (BPD) and/or mortality. Most commonly used NIV modes, including nasal continuous positive airway pressure, biphasic modes, such as Si-PAP or Bi-PAP, nasal intermittent positive pressure ventilation, high-flow nasal cannula, and newer NIV strategies, such as nasal high-frequency ventilation and noninvasive neurally adjusted ventilatory assist (NAVA), are discussed in this issue.

Retinopathy of prematurity (ROP) is one of the leading yet largely preventable causes of childhood blindness in the United States and worldwide. Since the mid-1940s, the history of O_2 use in newborn infants has been pretty intricate and inundated with misconceptions and errors and will continue to be so in 2023. As O_2 is a very potent drug often used inappropriately in the clinical environment; its administration needs to be improved in neonatal care. Tissue oxygenation is complex and depends on many factors other than pulse oximetry (SpO_2), including hemoglobin concentration and quality, cardiac output, peripheral vascular resistance, systemic blood flow, O_2 delivery, microcirculation, and others. Excess O_2 is a neonatal health hazard, and hyperoxemia should be prevented from the delivery room and throughout the hospital stay. This review focuses on the most current methods, evidence, and controversies in clinical practice regarding the basics of ROP and SpO_2 monitoring in neonates.

Pulse Oximetry (PO) is a widely available, simple, rapid, accurate, and noninvasive method of measuring blood O_2 levels (saturation), and the use of PO as a screen for critical congenital heart defects (CCHD) is based on the rationale that the majority of newborn babies with CCHD will have a degree of hypoxemia, many of which may be clinically undetectable. Pulse oximetry screening (POS) was first described over 20 years ago; however, in recent years major clinical trials have demonstrated consistent test accuracy for the detection of CCHD. International uptake of POS has progressed well over the last 10 years with most major high-income countries now recommending screening. Another review is presented that describes the evidence base that has led to this, the current debate regarding the choice of screening algorithm, and the future areas for further research.

Venous access is required by most acutely/critically ill neonates, especially those born preterm. Access is required for implementing management strategies, such as stabilization, medications, fluids, nutrition, and transfusion of blood products. However, achieving and maintaining venous access in these neonates can be difficult, especially in preterm infants. Their veins are small and fragile, coupled with physiologic immaturity that increases the risk of venous/capillary leakage. Many neonates may require vascular access for weeks or months, putting the neonate at risk for multiple attempts to obtain vascular access across time as well as complications.

Peripheral intravenous (PIV) catheters and peripherally inserted central catheters (PICC) are two common vascular access approaches used in the NICU and have traditionally been the most studied in the neonatal literature. PICCs offer a long-term solution for venous access in neonates due to their central placement and allow for the infusion of nutritional products, fluids, and medications that can be difficult on peripherally located veins due to fluid pH, osmolarity, or cytotoxicity. PIVs are intended for short-term needs and prove to be a challenge to access and maintain. Both options offer advantages and disadvantages. An alternative to PIVs and PICCs is the midline peripheral catheter, also referred to as an extended dwell PIV catheter, which is further described in this issue.

Innovative strategies are being developed to improve the long-term outcomes in high-risk infants. Novel studies are using breastmilk analysis aimed to optimize neurodevelopment in preterm infants. Years ago, the NICU was a very formula-based culture. Before commercial formula became widely available, infants who were not breastfed were generally fed evaporated milk with water and corn syrup. Now we are analyzing the nutritional composition of breastmilk and researching the use of individualized fortification of breastmilk for optimal growth and neurodevelopment of preterm infants in the NICU.

Mother's Own Milk (MOM) is known to decrease complications in preterm infants, and when unavailable, it is recommended that preterm very-low-birth-weight infants be fed donor human milk (DHM). Due to the pasteurization, processing, and lactation stage of donors, DHM does not contain the same nutritional, immunologic, and microbial components as MOM. Another review summarizes the differences between MOM and DHM, the potential effects on health outcomes, and the clinical implications of these differences. In addition, the acceptance of DHM by neonatal intensive care families and staff, the impact of DHM availability on MOM consumption, and the use of DHM in infants who are not preterm and very-low-birth-weight infants are reviewed. Implications for research and clinical practice are also discussed.

Telehealth, also referred to as telemedicine, is yet another innovative technology discussed in this issue of *Critical Care Nursing Clinics of North America* that has seen a surge in use during the last several years. Telehealth has proven to be a valuable and growing method of managing the neonatal population, including neonates and children with medical complexity. Telehealth helps support the transition from hospital to home, provides remote monitoring to neonates, and extends the reach of pediatric subspecialists with neonatal expertise to underserved and rural communities. Moreover, telehealth care models may address SDOH, increase equity, and reduce disparities by extending the reach of providers to underserved communities.

Our final article looks at Neonatal Nursing from a Global Perspective. Neonatal and maternal mortality rates are key indicators of a country's well-being and level of development. Every country has its own standards and protocols of care. Some countries provide better health care than others. Partnerships are very important for improving patient outcomes. By joining forces with other organizations, including interprofessional ones, partnerships amplify the efforts of an individual organization to improve the health of global society members. Organizing the neonatal nursing workforce and empowerment are vitally important for improving neonatal outcomes. The Council of International Neonatal Nurses, Inc (COINN) has been the only voice for global neonatal nurses and has worked on each global initiative, first by endorsing reports and then by attending United Nations meetings where the first *"Born Too Soon"* report was launched in 2012. Empowered nurses change practice. International organizations like COINN help local organizations to be involved at the global level and address their national needs appropriately. At this moment in time, leaders of civil society, policymakers, professional organizations, universities, ministries of health, and nursing councils are working together for a call to action to have a better-prepared workforce. Only when this becomes a reality will neonatal mortality globally decrease, and preventable death will be averted.

We hope that you enjoy Part I of this two-part issue dedicated to neonates and their families. Part II will include hot topics related to prenatal bonding, multidisciplinary perspectives of neuroprotective care for small babies, neonatal death, perceptions and current practices for neonatal pain, an update on new opioids, psychoactive drugs, synthetic marijuana, neonatal abstinence syndrome (NAS) and neonatal opioid withdrawal syndrome (NOWS), nonpharmacologic interventions for feeding success in NAS/NOWS babies, nurse-led telehealth interventions, family-centered care, palliative care and/or end-of-life care, and legacy building through the use of heartbeat recordings embedded in music and more.

Leslie Altimier, DNP, RN, NE-BC, MSN, BSN
Cardinal Glennon Children's Hospital
1465 South Grand Avenue
St. Louis, MO 63104, USA

E-mail address:
laltimier@gmail.com

Dangerous Things We Used to Do in Neonatology

Catherine Lewis Witt, PhD, NNP-BC

KEYWORDS

- Neonatology • Neonatal care • History • Respiratory care • Medications
- Thermoregulation

KEY POINTS

- A lack of knowledge can lead to ineffective care and medical errors.
- A review of evidence is important before beginning any new treatment.
- Openness to ongoing learning is essential in neonatal care.

INTRODUCTION

In 1903, Martin Couney opened an infant incubator show at Coney Island, New York. This exhibition of premature infants continued for 40 years, allowing visitors to marvel at tiny infants being cared for with emerging technology. Although we are rightly appalled at the idea of neonates being placed on public display, we must also acknowledge the role of skilled nurses who were largely unnamed and underappreciated. These nurses provided treatments, care, and feeding to the infants and recorded weights, feeding amounts, and other events that occurred during their care. The observations they made and the notes they kept contributed significantly to the early progress of neonatal intensive care.[1]

Those who cared for premature and ill newborns as neonatal intensive care units (NICUs) were developed were, in general, consciences, professional staff dedicated to providing the best possible care. It is easy to criticize what was done in the past. However, we must not forget that even some of our best care today may later be determined misguided or even dangerous. Future generations may look at the care we provide now and wonder what we were thinking. Therefore, it is important to approach all we do with humility, a desire to learn, and the willingness to admit when we make mistakes. This article looks back on practices that, though considered best at the time, we now know were unadvisable and sometimes dangerous.

Loretto Heights School of Nursing, Regis University, 3333 Regis Boulevard, Mail Code G-8, Denver, CO 80221, USA
E-mail address: cwitt@regis.edu

Crit Care Nurs Clin N Am 36 (2024) 1–10
https://doi.org/10.1016/j.cnc.2023.08.003
ccnursing.theclinics.com

THERMOREGULATION

The importance of keeping the preterm infant warm has been known since the 1800s. Early incubators were used in exhibits at World's Fairs, Coney Island displays, and at other exhibitions. Understanding of heat balance, methods of heat loss, and brown fat metabolism increased during the 1950s and 1960s.[2,3] Early incubators were heated with hot water running from a boiler on the outside through a pipe that ran underneath the bed. Later incubators used fans to circulate heat, which increased the noise level both inside and outside the incubator.

Rectal temperatures were recommended for all term and preterm infants when admitted to the nursery or the NICU. The goal was to rule out an imperforate anus as well as obtain an admission temperature. This practice continued for many years despite risks of trauma to the intestinal mucosa.[4]

Despite increased knowledge and improved incubators, mishaps occurred with heat lamps, water bottles, and warming packs. Reports of iatrogenic burns in hospitalized newborns have been recorded as recently as 2022, usually due to inappropriate water temperature or the use of warming devices.[5] Before the development of commercial heel warmers, warm washcloths were often used to warm the heel before blood sampling. Instances of warming the wet washcloth in the microwave were reported, resulting in burns to the skin. Hot compresses to relieve perceived abdominal pain or "colic" also resulted in reports of scalding or more serious injury. A description of early neonatal transport describes using a light bulb for warming the transport incubator and supplementing it with hot water bottles, taking care to avoid direct contact with the infant.[6] Heat lamps were also used for wound healing and diaper rash, in the belief that heat and light would dry the wound and accelerate healing. Before the availability of pulse oximetry, burns occurred from the measurement of transcutaneous oxygen, which required a heated electrode that had to be moved every few hours to avoid injuring the skin.

NUTRITION

Feeding the preterm neonate was considered as essential as keeping the baby warm. Although the benefits of maternal milk were recognized as early as the 1800s, feeding practices for term and preterm infants did not always reflect this knowledge.[7]

A nursing state board preparation book from 1942 directs nurses to allow term infants to breastfeed for a maximum time of 3 to 5 minutes, but not until 6 to 8 hours after birth and then every 4 to 8 hours. Each breastfeeding was to be followed with "5% lactose solution ½ to 1 ounce." A preterm infant was to be fed evaporated milk every 3 hours.[8]

Before commercial formula became widely available, infants who were not breastfed were generally fed evaporated milk with water and corn syrup. In the 1950s, premature infants were noted to grow better with increased protein. This led to oral feedings or parenteral nutrition with a high-protein content, sometimes leading to fluid retention and metabolic acidosis.[9] Preterm infants were often limited in fluids, both feedings and intravenous (IV) fluids, for the first 72 hours or so due to the presence of "edema" and concern for respiratory distress.[9]

The introduction of enteral feedings varied significantly and progressed as knowledge of optimal growth, gastrointestinal maturity, and nutritional impact improved. As recently as the 1970s, it was thought that preterm neonates less than 1500 g should not be fed for the first 48 hours and that feeding should begin with 5% or 10% glucose water for the first one or two feedings in case of aspiration.[10] Because indwelling oral gastric tubes were not available, gavage tubes were placed for each feeding (every 1 to 3 hours). The feeding flowed by gravity for more than 10 to 20 minutes (never by syringe pressure) and the feeding tube was removed at the end of the feeding. Feedings were generally withheld from neonates requiring assisted ventilation until they were in a recovery phase or requiring "less oxygen," an arbitrary number that might mean less than 40% oxygen or some other standard.[10]

Parenteral nutrition was limited in the 1970s and early 1980s and was mostly limited to glucose infusions with electrolytes added on day 2 or 3. Early IV protein was usually provided with casein or fibrin hydrolysates, but these were often poorly tolerated by the neonate.[9] Hyperalimentation was often not started for several days, and then only if it was anticipated the neonate would not be able to receive feedings for 7 to 10 days. Amino acid formulas were introduced in the 1990s, and trace elements, vitamins, and intralipids were added to make a more complete preparation. The importance of early nutritional support and the need for amino acids immediately after birth in the preterm infant was not recognized until the 2000s. Consequently, feeding practices varied widely among units and regions of the country.[11]

RESPIRATORY CARE

Instructions for nurses caring for the preterm neonate in 1942 included these directions: "Provide 10% carbon dioxide and 90% oxygen TID for 3 minutes for the first 3 days."[8] From the 1950s into the 1960s, oxygen was recognized as a treatment for respiratory distress in the preterm infant. Still, a lack of guidelines about appropriate oxygen levels meant that excessive or inconsistent amounts of oxygen were often provided. The most common method of administration was to infuse the oxygen directly into the incubator, which also resulted in significant swings in oxygen levels when the neonate was accessed through the portholes or an open incubator door. This practice, along with a lack of ability to easily monitor blood oxygen levels, resulted in increasing incidences of retinopathy of prematurity. As neonatal care progressed, oxygen hoods became more common and allowed for easier regulation of Fio_2. Until the advent of pulse oximetry and transcutaneous oxygen monitoring, frequent blood gases were the only way to determine the neonate's oxygen level. If an umbilical catheter was unavailable, then radial or brachial punctures were used.[12] The use of umbilical catheters made frequent monitoring of arterial blood gases more practical.

Mechanical ventilation for preterm neonates was not widely available until the mid-1960s. In 1964, President John F Kennedy's son died at 34 weeks gestation, likely due to respiratory distress syndrome. This led to increased funding for preterm care and the treatment of respiratory diseases.[9] It was recognized by the 1970s that preterm lung disease was characterized by decreased surfactant, increased alveolar surface tension, and decreased lung compliance. Pulmonary vasoconstriction was also recognized as a contributing factor.[12] It was noted by these authors in 1973 that it was important to keep the neonate warm and well-oxygenated and to limit $NaHCO_3$ administration to every 4 to 6 hours.

Pneumothorax was frequently treated by placing the neonate in 100% oxygen via hood in the hopes that this would enhance the reabsorption rate of the air from the pleural cavity (nitrogen washout). It was thought that the inhalation of 100% oxygen would decrease the partial pressure of nitrogen in the alveolus. This would cause the nitrogen to diffuse from the pleural space into the alveoli with faster resolution of the pneumothorax.[13]

Continuous positive airway pressure (CPAP) or positive pressure ventilation were the primary types of assisted ventilation available in the 1970s to early 1980s. CPAP was initiated if the oxygen requirement increased over .70 Fio_2.[14] Most CPAP was delivered via an endotracheal tube. Nasal CPAP was also used beginning in the 1970s. Continuous airway pressure of up to 12 cm H_2O was used as needed to lower the oxygen requirement.[14]

Positive pressure ventilation was the most commonly used ventilator in the 1970s, although negative pressure devices were also being tried around that time. Volume ventilation was also available in some places. Nasal insertion of the endotracheal tube was most often used. The rate on the commonly used Baby Bird ventilator was set by adjusting the expiratory time. The high pressures and rates sometimes needed to oxygenate a neonate with surfactant deficiency resulted in frequent air leaks and barotrauma, contributing to bronchopulmonary dysplasia (BPD) and pulmonary interstitial emphysema. Neonates were weaned from the ventilator by gradually decreasing the pressure or ventilator rate until only positive end-expiratory pressure was left. The infant was usually left on endotracheal CPAP for some time before extubating.[14]

Routine chest physiotherapy (CPT), either by percussion or vibration, was done for most ventilated neonates. This was thought to loosen secretions and prevent atelectasis. Endotracheal suctioning accompanied this, often with the instillation of normal saline to loosen secretions. CPT was used in the delivery room in some facilities. The intent was to clear lung secretions or to improve ventilation, despite no evidence to support this practice.

Apnea was noted to be a common occurrence in preterm infants, illustrating the need for continuous cardiac monitoring. Before the development of hydrogel, EKG electrodes consisted of subdermal needles inserted under the skin of the chest. Apnea was treated by pulling a string tied to the infant's foot and pulling on from outside the incubator or other noxious practices such as bouncing the mattress under the neonate. Apnea was sometimes treated with aminophylline, which had a narrow therapeutic window, requiring monitoring of levels on a regular basis.

RESUSCITATION

In the 1940s, instructions for neonatal resuscitation included "compression of the chest 20 times a minute" or "folding and unfolding the infant like a book to produce intermittent compression of the chest."[8] These instructions included taking care to avoid trauma! Over time, various methods were tried, including a 1950s positive pressure air lock chamber that cycled times of high pressure with that of no pressure in hopes of inducing gasping with each cycle of decreased pressure. Oxygen was included in the chamber as it was thought to be absorbed through the skin also into the lungs when a breath occurred. Other options suggested immersion in cold water, use of aromatic spirits of ammonia, insufflation of oxygen into the stomach, and even the use of bellows connected to a bulb inserted in the upper airway that blew air into the lungs.[9,15,16]

In 1953, Virginia Apgar published her method of assessing the neonate at birth. This led to increased attention to the needs of the neonate in the delivery room and the need to improve care. In 1958, a self-inflating bag-mask unit was developed to provide oxygen or room air directly through a face mask and allow for rescue breathing.[9,17]

The American Heart Association and the American Academy of Pediatrics (AAP) began to develop education for community hospitals with the aim of improving newborn care. This program, which was called the Neonatal Education Program, became the basis for the Neonatal Resuscitation Program, which was introduced in 1987.[15,18] This program standardized neonatal resuscitation and continues ongoing research and refinement of recommendations.

Some recommendations have changed significantly over the years: regarding medications in the delivery room, the use of oxygen, and the approach to meconium-stained amniotic fluid. NaHCO$_3$ went from a relatively routine recommended medication to only use if good evidence for acidosis to not recommended at all as part of resuscitation. Volume infusion changed from 5% albumin to normal saline, then to much more judicious use with evidence of volume depletion. Narcan is also rarely used now, and the dose of epinephrine changed over the years. Oxygen recommendations went from 100% oxygen to a more targeted approach, using pulse oximetry and evaluating the neonate's response.[18]

Meconium aspiration, as a contributor to lung disease, was thought best treated through prevention. Neonates born through meconium-stained fluid, particularly thick, particulate meconium, were suctioned on the perineum to clear the mouth and nose before delivery of the shoulders and presumably the first breath. The goal was to avoid meconium being aspirated from the pharynx with the onset of respirations. DeLee suction catheters with mucus traps were used. The early DeLee catheters had one catheter equipped with a mouthpiece that the clinician used like a straw to pull fluid from the other catheter into a small canister or trap. This required someone to be near enough to the perineum to reach one end of the catheter into the neonate's mouth and nose and suck on the other catheter.

Once delivered, neonates with meconium-stained fluid were to be intubated, and the trachea suctioned to eliminate any trace of meconium found below the vocal cords. Ideally, this would happen before the onset of regular respirations and could be repeated more than once if meconium was found. Once this was completed, the neonate could be stimulated or ventilated as needed. This was later changed to intubate only non-vigorous neonates or those with thick meconium. This procedure is no longer recommended.[16,18]

PHARMACOLOGY

Perhaps no area of neonatal care has more lessons to learn than the use of medications. Several medications in the NICU were either used in incorrect doses, without good evidence or not used at all.

Vitamin K

Hemorrhagic disease of the newborn was first described in 1894, and the relationship between neonatal hemorrhage and prothrombin deficiency was demonstrated in 1932.[19,20] The role of vitamin K in the prevention of hemorrhagic disease of the newborn became known in 1939, and the prophylactic use of vitamin K began in the 1940s. In 1954, the AAP recommended newborns receive a dose of 5 mg.[21] Later doses of up to 10 mg daily for 3 days were used, especially in neonates who were not feeding.[19,20] Some infants received cumulative doses of over 50 mg. Increased incidences of hyperbilirubinemia and kernicterus were reported, and in 1961, the AAP revised their recommendations to 0.5 to 1 mg parenterally.[21]

Hexachlorophene

Although technically not a medication, the concern for infection led to increased efforts to eradicate common organisms such as *Staphylococcus aureus* from the nursery. Neonates were bathed with 3% hexachlorophene (HCP) soap on admission and then every 2 to 3 days during their stay. The solution was sometimes used to clean incubators, other equipment, and hospital laundries. HCP was also used in lotions, cosmetics, baby talcum powder, and antiseptic solutions. These products were also used on neonatal skin. Reports of seizures and abnormal neurologic activity were reported during the 1960s, and the practice was discontinued in the early 1970s.[20,22]

Epsom Salts Enemas

Fortunately, a short-lived practice, the use of Epsom salt enemas on neonates with respiratory distress syndrome was thought to decrease the edema and excess water contributing to the disease. Symptoms of magnesium toxicity and hypocalcemia resulted in this practice being discontinued by 1975.[22]

Benzyl alcohol

Benzyl alcohol was used as a preservative in many multiuse medication vials. It was sometimes present in normal saline solutions used to flush umbilical catheters and could, in those instances, be administered several times a day. The metabolite of benzyl alcohol is benzoate, which is known to displace bilirubin from albumin.[23] Neonates were reported to demonstrate metabolic acidosis, "gasping syndrome," renal failure, and neurologic symptoms. The Food and Drug Administration (FDA) recommended that benzyl alcohol should be discontinued as a preservative in 1982.[20,23]

Intravenous Vitamin E

In 1949, Owens and Owens postulated that retrolental fibroplasia (RLF), now known as retinopathy of prematurity) was related to vitamin E deficiency.[20,23] Although evidence that vitamin E supplementation was sparse, many units added oral vitamin E to feedings. Because many preterm infants were not fed for extended periods, an IV solution (E-Ferol Injection) was developed in 1983. Soon after, neonates developed hepatomegaly, thrombocytopenia, jaundice, ascites, and azotemia. These symptoms were likely due to the polysorbate used as a solubilizer. After the deaths of at least 40 infants, the drug was recalled less than 6 months after it was introduced.[20,23]

Antibiotics

Until recent efforts toward antibiotic stewardship, concern for sepsis meant that most neonates admitted to an NICU were treated prophylactically with antimicrobials. *Staphylococcus aureus* and *group B streptococcus* were common infective agents. Penicillin became available in the 1940s, and penicillin-resistant staph aureus was beginning to be seen in the 1950s. In 1953, sulfisoxazole, a sulfonamide, was introduced. Because it required less frequent dosing, it was readily accepted as an alternative or adjunct to penicillin. By 1959, it was recognized that an increased mortality rate and an increased rate of kernicterus could be attributed to the use of the sulfonamide due to competition with bilirubin for albumin binding sites.[20,22]

In the 1950s, chloramphenicol was also used for prophylaxis due to its broad effectiveness for gram-positive and gram-negative organisms. In 1958, it was reported that neonates receiving large doses of chloramphenicol developed abdominal distension, pallid cyanosis ("gray baby syndrome"), and cardiovascular collapse. The recommended dosage was decreased, and soon after, in 1960, its use in neonates was discontinued.[22]

Steroids

Owing to the prolonged use of mechanical ventilation and oxygen and the high pressures sometimes used with early ventilators, BPD was a frequent complication in preterm neonates. This was particularly problematic before the use of exogenous surfactants. Dexamethasone caused a rapid improvement in oxygen requirement and in lung function, allowing neonates to be more readily weaned from mechanical ventilation. Although the anti-inflammatory benefits of dexamethasone certainly worked in decreasing ventilator time, the long-term adverse effects such as neuromotor impairment, increased risk for cerebral palsy, and poor growth made the routine, long-term use of steroids unadvisable. Safe dosages and length of treatment in neonates with BPD are still being studied and should be used with caution.[23,24]

Pain Relief

Until the 1980s, it was thought that preterm neonates either did not feel pain or did not respond to pain in the same way due to their immature nervous system. In addition, the fear of respiratory depression in a neonate with respiratory compromise limited the use of opioids or other pain medications.[25] Consequently, most neonates were significantly undertreated for pain, including for surgical procedures. Paralytic agents were often used without accompanying pain relief or sedation. Perceived simple procedures such as heel sticks, venipuncture, or arterial blood sampling were not accompanied by efforts toward pain control. Even procedures such as intubation, ophthalmology examinations, or lumbar punctures were not considered painful enough to require treatment. Studies reporting the consequences of repetitive and unrelieved pain emerged in the 1990s and 2000s along with instruments designed to assess neonatal pain. Despite the growing body of evidence, neonatal pain is not always well recognized and treated, even today.[26]

Sedation was more readily used, likely due to less fear around respiratory distress. However, the risks of sedatives in the neonate were not clearly understood. Chloral hydrate was commonly used in the 1980s and 1990s without understanding of the cumulative effects on the neonate.

DEVELOPMENTAL AND FAMILY-CENTERED CARE

In 1934, a set of identical quintuplets was born in a farmhouse in rural Ontario, Canada. The girls who were 2 months premature were initially quarantined in a parlor in the farmhouse and cared for by nurses brought in to help. Their mother was only allowed limited contact. She could look at them through the door but was not allowed to hold or touch them due to concerns about infections. At 2 to 3 months of age, the quintuplets were moved to a separate building next to their family home. There, they lived for the next 8 years with their parents and siblings having limited visitation or interaction. However; the public could visit "Quintland", a popular tourist attraction. Visitors could watch the girls play through windows looking into the nursery or observe them in the playground attached to the building.[27] The quintuples were reunited with their parents and siblings at the age of 9 years, a process that unsurprisingly did not go well.

Those infants cared for in an incubator exhibit such as that on Coney Island, also suffered from a lack of parental interaction. Although mothers were allowed to visit, they were not allowed to participate in caring for their infants. There were some challenges when it was time for the infants to be discharged. Parents sometimes could not be located or were reluctant to assume care of their babies.[28]

As births moved into the hospital, parent interaction remained limited, even for full-term infants. Instructions to mothers from a hospital in 1963 list the times infants would be brought out to the mothers for feeding. No visitors were allowed, and one strange directive stated that the mother should not to unwrap the baby. Fathers could see the babies through the nursery window at prescribed times.[29] In the 1960s and 1970s, consumer demand led to a more family-centered approach to childbirth and infant care, at least for term infants.[29,30]

In the NICU, concern for infection limited the interaction of parents. Parents were considered "visitors," and strict schedules around feedings and other activities limited flexibility around parenting activities. When parents were allowed to visit, they were often required to wear gowns, gloves, and masks. Research into maternal bonding and attachment in the 1970s helped illustrate the difficulties faced by families due to prolonged separation from their infants. It was realized that early involvement in caring for the infant led to better caretaking behaviors and confidence on discharge. The development of private rooms for NICU babies has increased the ability of parents and other family members to spend time with their infant and learn caregiving skills.

Research into developmental care began to be documented in the 1980s. Before that, most NICUs consisted of large rooms, brightly lit, with little consideration for space or noise levels. Neonates who required mechanical ventilation were cared for on open radiant warmers with minimal protection from overwhelming levels of environmental and social stimulation.[29,30] Knowledge of preterm neonate behaviors was minimal. It was assumed, for instance, that preterm infants had little or no visual acuity and had minimal ability to interact with their environment. Little attention was paid to positioning while on mechanical ventilation, other than restraints to limit the possibility of accidental extubation.[29,30] Allowing a parent to hold an intubated neonate was forbidden for fear of accidental extubation. Even after the neonate was moved to an incubator or crib, simple positioning with blanket rolls, nests, or swaddling was not considered. Neonates were not protected from continuous bright lights or ambient noise. Although this has improved over the years, developmental care still needs to be applied somemore consistently and parents are sometimes thought of as visitors rather than part of the care team. Physical environments are slightly improved with single-family rooms, but improvement can still be made in most NICUs.

SUMMARY

There have been many improvements in neonatal care, especially since the early NICUs of the 1970s and 1980s. It is easy to look back and be proud of how well we are currently doing. Evidence-based care is considered an essential part of health care practices. We have worked hard to improve family-centered and developmental care, although room for improvement still exists. Significant progress in the ventilation of neonates has been seen. However, the lessons of our history illustrate we should not become complacent. Many of the practices described here were done because they were considered state-of-the-art at the time. It is important to remain humble and remember that in 40 years, much of what we do today might be included in an article such as this.

CLINICS CARE POINTS

- Learning from our past mistakes is a vital part of improving future care.
- Treatments and medications should not be introduced in the NICU without a careful review of the evidence supporting the intervention.
- Humility is essential in all areas of nursing and medicine. We are constantly learning new things.
- We should remember that much of what we do may later be discovered to be incorrect.

DISCLOSURE

The author has no financial or commercial conflicts of interest to disclose. The author has received no funding for the development of this article.

REFERENCES

1. Prescott S, Hehman MC. Premature infant care in the early 20th century. J Obstet Gynecol Neonatal Nurs 2017;46:637–46.
2. Silverman WA, Fertig JW, Berger AP. The influence of the thermal environment upon the survival of newly born premature infants. Pediatrics 1958;22:876–86.
3. Raju TNK. Growth of neonatal perinatal medicine – a historical perspective. In: Martin RJ, Fanaroff AA, Walsh MC, editors. Fanaroff and martin's neonatal-perinatal medicine. 11th edition. PA: Elsevier; 2020. p. 2–17.
4. Agren J. Thermal environment of the intensive care nursery. In: Martin RJ, Fanaroff AA, Walsh MC, editors. Fanaroff and martin's neonatal-perinatal medi-cine. 11th edition. Philadelphia: Elsevier; 2020. p. 566–76.
5. Muntean A, Stoica I, Enescu DM. Etiology of neonatal burns: a systemic review. Ann Burns Fire Disasters 2022;35:186–93.
6. Losty MA, Orlofsky I, Wallace HM. A transport service for premature babies. Am J Nurs 1950;50:10–2.
7. Dowling D. Lessons from the past: a brief history of the influence of social, eco-nomic, and scientific factors on infant feeding. Newborn Infant Nurs Rev 2005; 5(1):2–9.
8. Cowan CM. Obstetric and gynecologic nursing. In: Butzerin EB, et al, editors. State board questions and answers for nurses. 20th edition. Philadelphia: Lippin-cott; 1942. p. 697–828.
9. Philip AGS. The evolution of neonatology. Pediatr Res 2005;58:799–815.
10. Fanaroff A, Klaus M. Feeding the low-birth-weight infant. In: Klaus M, Fanaroff A, editors. Care of the high-risk neonate. Philadelphia: WB Saunders; 1973. p. 77–89.
11. Poindexter BB, Martin CR. Nutrient requirements/nutritional support in premature neonates. In: Martin RJ, Fanaroff AA, Walsh MC, editors. Fanaroff and martin's neonatal-perinatal medicine. 11th edition. Philadelphia: Elsevier; 2020. p. 670–89.
12. Klaus M, Fanaroff A. Respiratory problems. In: Klaus M, Fanaroff A, editors. Care of the high-risk neonate. Philadelphia: WB Saunders; 1973. p. 119–51.
13. Shaireen H, Rabi Y, Metcalfe A, et al. Impact of oxygen concentration on time to resolution of spontaneous pneumothorax in term infants: a population-based cohort study. BMC Pediatr 2014;28. https://doi.org/10.1186/1471-2431-14-208.
14. Llewellyn A, Swyer P. Assisted ventilation. In: Klaus M, Fanaroff A, editors. Care of the high-risk neonate. Philadelphia: WB Saunders; 1973. p. 152–67.
15. Zaichkin J, Wiswell TE. The history of neonatal resuscitation. Neonatal Network 2002;21(f):21–8.
16. O'Donnell CPF, Gibson AT, Davis PG. Pinching, electrocution, ravens' beaks, and positive pressure ventilation: a brief history of neonatal resuscitation. Arch Dis Child Fetal Neonatal Ed 2006;92:F369–73.
17. Apgar V, Holaday DA, James LS, et al. Evaluation of the newborn infant-second report. JAMA 1958;168:1985–8.
18. American Academy of Pediatrics, American Heart Association. In: Weiner GM, editor. Textbook of neonatal resuscitation. 8th edition. Itasca, IL: AAP; 2021.

19. Robertson AF. Reflections on errors in neonatology: I. The "hands-off" years, 1920 – 1950. J Perinatol 2003;23:48–55.
20. Lussky RC, Cifuentes RF, Siddappa AM. A history of neonatal medicine- past accomplishments, lessons learned, and future challenges, part 1, the first century. J Pediatr Pharmacol Ther 2005;10:76–89.
21. American Academy of Pediatrics, Committee on Fetus and Newborn. Standards and recommendations for hospital care of newborn infants. 2nd edition. Evanston: American Academy of Pediatrics; 1954.
22. Robertson AF. Reflections on errors in neonatology: II. The "heroic" years, 1950 – 1970. J Perinatol 2003;23:154–61.
23. Robertson AF. Reflections on errors in neonatology: III. The "experienced" years, 1970-2000. J Perinatol 2003;23:240–9.
24. American Academy of Pediatrics. Postnatal corticosteroids to prevent or treat chronic lung disease following preterm birth. Pediatrics 2022;149(6).
25. Donato J, Rao K, Lewis T. Pharmacology of common analgesic and sedative drugs used in the neonatal intensive care. Clin Perinatol 2019;46:673–92.
26. Walden M. Pain assessment and management. In: Verklan MT, Walden M, Forest S, editors. Core curriculum for neonatal intensive care nursing. 6th edition. Philadelphia: Elsevier; 2021. p. 270–87.
27. Thomas LM. The changing role of parents in neonatal care: a historical review. Neonatal Network 2008;2:91–100.
28. Memorial Hospital Colorado Springs. Information for mothers, 1963.
29. Davis L, Mohay H, Edwards H. Mothers' involvement in caring for their preterm infants: an historical overview. J Adv Nurs 2003;42:578–86.
30. Jaeger CB, Browne JV. The science. In: Kenner C, McGrath JM, editors. Developmental care of newborns and infants: a guide for health professionals. 3rd edition. Philadelphia: Wolters Kluwer; 2023. p. 1–18.

The Effects of Health Disparities on Neonatal Outcomes

Erin J. Mays, MSN, APRN, NNP-BC[a],*, Stephanie Diggs, MD[b],
Zachary A. Vesoulis, MD, MS[b], Barbara Warner, MD, MS[b]

KEYWORDS

- Health disparities • Prematurity • Infant mortality • Breastfeeding
- Family experience • Institutional racism • Structural racism

KEY POINTS

- The first step in dismantling health disparities is acknowledging the presence of deeply embedded racism and its long-standing impact on health care in minority populations.
- Black infants are more likely to be born premature and are at a higher risk for neonatal morbidities such as intraventricular hemorrhage and necrotizing enterocolitis.
- Discrimination and segregation in neighborhoods have led to poor access and/or poor-quality care in Black communities.
- Cultural implications should be considered when looking at why breastfeeding initiation, continuation, and discharge rates are lower for Black infants.
- Attention should be paid to the lack of diversity in the health care field and how it affects patient outcomes.

INTRODUCTION

Imagine that there were two infants born at the same gestational age but with very different outcomes. Baby A was born at 28 weeks gestation, admitted to the newborn intensive care unit (NICU) on bubble continuous positive airway pressure (BCPAP), required respiratory support until 32 weeks gestation, and then discharged home at 39 weeks to mom with no complications. Baby B was also born at 28 weeks gestation and admitted to the NICU on BCPAP, but respiratory support was escalated with intubation and mechanical ventilation until 38 weeks and room air maintenance occurred at 45 weeks. Around 29 weeks, Baby B developed necrotizing enterocolitis (NEC); in addition, the 10 days of life head ultrasound results showed

[a] St. Louis Children's Hospital NICU, 1 Childrens Place, St Louis, MO 63110, USA; [b] Division of Newborn Medicine, Department of Pediatrics, Washington University School of Medicine, 1 Childrens Place, #8116-NWT 8, St Louis, MO 63110, USA
* Corresponding author.
E-mail address: erin.mays@bjc.org

Crit Care Nurs Clin N Am 36 (2024) 11–22
https://doi.org/10.1016/j.cnc.2023.08.006
ccnursing.theclinics.com

the development of an intraventricular hemorrhage (IVH). At 43 weeks, despite signs of oral readiness, progression toward full oral feeding was unsuccessful, and the infant required placement of a gastrointestinal tube the week before final discharge home with mom at 48 weeks. Are you wondering why these infants had such different hospital courses? One obvious difference is Baby A was born to a White mother, and Baby B was born to a Black mother. This unfortunate scenario plays out in many NICUs across the United States every day despite all the advancements made in neonatology. How does race impact the outcome of these infants? What can we do to improve these outcomes? Where, when, and why did the difference in outcomes begin?

Disparities begin to impact children even before they are born, primarily through differences in prematurity and mortality. In the United States, 10.5% of infants are born prematurely every year, and this continues to increase at a steady pace over the last few years despite continuous advancements in all areas of medicine. Black women are 52% more likely than all other women to have premature babies, which is defined as birth before 37 weeks gestation. The estimates of prematurity among babies born to Black women range between 7.3% and 24.0%.[1] A major contributor to the high-rate of prematurity among Black women is a lack of adequate prenatal care[2] and is defined as receiving prenatal care after 20 weeks gestation or receiving less than 50% of the suggested prenatal visits.[3] In at least one estimate, Black women are more than twice as likely as non-Hispanic White women to receive no prenatal care during pregnancy.[4] In a meta-analysis of 19 studies covering more than 600,000 women, Black women were found to consistently have delayed access to prenatal care, an effect strongly influenced by the degree of segregation present in the community.[5] Prematurity negatively impacts most of the major organ systems, which can result in adverse outcomes for these infants.[6]

The disparities in outcomes evident in the example above have roots that started well before admission to the NICU. Roots related to resource allocation resulting from structural racism. The United States has a long-standing history of institutional and structural racism, with roots in slavery but persisting and continuing to influence clinical practice even in the twenty-first century. It has been so embedded in the fabric of our society that it is often committed automatically and unconsciously by those who are not victims of it. Interpersonal racism is enhanced or reinforced by institutional racism, societal structures of policy, laws, and customs, which implicitly or explicitly disenfranchise minorities.[7] Examples of structural racism include the segregation of schools and voter suppression laws. Viewed through an epidemiologic lens, the American Medical Association refers to structural racism as the way society promotes discrimination through housing, employment, health care, and other systems that impact the delivery of resources to minorities.[8] The scarcity of affordable housing in minority communities is a result of structural racism. It is not surprising that a lack of resources has led to a plethora of health disparities and preventable differences in disease processes that are experienced by disadvantaged racial and ethnic groups of people.[9]

Disparities continue to impact neonates after birth, as Black infants frequently receive care in hospitals that lack quality resources.[10] As with most disparities, this problem exists as a consequence of structural racism, in this case, the 1933 establishment of the Home Owners' Loan Corporation (HOLC).[11] This quasi-governmental agency was created as a part of Roosevelt's New Deal with the intention of stabilizing foreclosures during the Great Depression through favorable refinancing and government-sponsored origination of home loans. As a part of the underwriting process, the default risk of individual loans was color-coded by geographic location (with red representing the highest risk). Although officially intended as a measure to prevent high default rates, the pervasive racism of HOLC policymakers and appraisers led to the systematic coding of communities with high Black populations entirely in red, an action later termed "redlining." This not only kept Blacks from owning homes, but it also kept resources out of predominately Black neighborhoods.[11] Although the HOLC was closed in 1954, the effects of redlining can still be seen on maps more than 70 years later with less tree canopy,[12] higher vacancy rates, a greater proportion of rented versus owned property,[13] and lower property values in formerly red-lined areas.[14] This resulted in poorer neighborhoods with inferior education and inadequate health care.[15] The lack of health care in these neighborhoods led to a higher incidence of chronic conditions such as diabetes, hypertension, and addiction. These conditions greatly impact women and their unborn children before pregnancy.[6]

As an additional effect of redlining, funds for technology, supplies, and equipment were diverted to hospitals in predominantly White neighborhoods. Even in urban settings with tertiary care centers, inadequate public transportation systems still restrict minorities from accessing higher quality health care in other neighborhoods, relegating them to local subpar services. Although the official act of redlining was terminated in 1968 with the passage of the Fair Housing Act, the impacts on health care continue to manifest today with greater adverse outcomes in hospitals that serve a patient population that is greater than 35% Black. This can be contributed to the quality of care.[10] These hospitals frequently have a lack of resources available for patients and staff. They are usually understaffed with nurses, resulting in unsafe assignments. This can cause insufficient use of best evidence-based practices and policies further leading to subpar care.[15] It also increases the risk of higher infection rates that then impact the mortality rate for at-risk infants. A recent retrospective study by Lui and colleagues of more than 20,000 premature infants (22–29 weeks gestation) that weighed between 401 and 1500 g at birth from 135 NICUs in California found that Black infants were more likely to receive care in hospitals with a higher rate of hospital-acquired infections. Although the reasons for these rates were not identified, they may be attributed to fewer resources and inadequate staffing.[16]

Informal racial segregation still exists today; red lines are no longer present on the maps, but it is easy to see where they once were by the demographics of the neighborhoods. In major metropolitan cities, including Chicago, Detroit, New York, and St Louis, segregation persists—Black people live in what is deemed as "Black neighborhoods" and Whites live in "White neighborhoods" which closely follow the same geographic boundaries established by HOLC almost 100 years ago. Although this practice provided privileges and benefits for White people, it had the opposite effect on Blacks. Minority communities often have lower wage jobs and are plagued with higher crime rates and destitute circumstances instead of high-paying jobs and an abundance of resources.[17] Residents of these communities also have a shorter life expectancy of 5 years.[18]

Evidence suggests that racial disparities correlate with the quality of the NICU where infants receive care but also that Black infants are more likely to receive lower quality care in any NICU.[19] Although Black women are more likely to live closer to a high-level NICU, White women are more likely to deliver there. The reason for this has not been clearly defined but is thought to be due to insurance restrictions.[20] This trend of restricted and lower access to care occurs across all regions of the United States[20] and is another example of structural racism leading to racial disparities. These disparities can lead to increased risk for morbidities and mortality, lower breastfeeding rates, and negative family experiences.[15]

MORTALITY

The increased incidence of prematurity among Black mothers means that a disproportionate burden of adverse outcomes, including complications of prematurity and death, falls on these same mothers. The United States has the highest infant mortality rate (IMR), defined as death within the first year of life, of any upper-income country. The national average mortality rate in the United States is 5.4 per 1000 live births, 37% higher than in neighboring Canada. It is not surprising, given the higher incidence of morbidities among Black infants, that the mortality rate for these infants would also be higher. Infant mortality is not evenly distributed by race; infants born to White mothers have a rate below the national average at 4.6 per 1000 live births, whereas infants born to Black mothers have double the IMR at 10.8 per 1000 live births.[3] Although these rates have been decreasing over time for all infants, rates for Black patients remain high, as do morbidities such as impaired neurodevelopment.[21] These effects are particularly acute for extremely low birth weight (defined as birth before 32 weeks gestation) infants who are at proportionately higher risk for adverse outcomes; any additional barriers to adequate health care from structural racism only exacerbate risks.[22]

The maternal vulnerability index (MVI) is a key predictor of mortality rates. This national index was developed by March of Dimes and Surgo Ventures in 2021 to look at key health aspects including those of physical health, mental health, reproductive health, substance abuse, and socioeconomic and environmental factors. It is used to determine areas where women are more vulnerable, which may translate into a greater risk of adverse outcomes for themselves and their infants.[3] There have yet to be any studies published using this index; however, the report produced by Surgo Ventures in 2022 breaks the United States into regions and shows that although the South has the highest maternal vulnerability, the Midwest has the most significant racial divide between Black and White mothers.[23] Using tools such as the MVI, health care providers can target Black women with high degrees of vulnerability, those at greatest risk of premature birth, and the ensuing complications. A reduction in premature delivery among Black mothers will directly translate into a reduction in infant mortality.[24] Given this direct correlation between premature birth, morbidities, and infant mortality,[25] it is imperative to not only recognize but also act to change clinical practice to begin improving these outcomes.

INTRAVENTRICULAR HEMORRHAGE

Returning to the case of Baby B, we saw the radiographic evidence of IVH at 10 days of life (29 weeks). IVH is a common form of brain injury in preterm infants and results from the rupture of the fragile vessels in the germinal matrix. IVH risk increases with decreasing gestational age and birth weight,[26] increasing degree of hypoxia,[27] or significant hemodynamic compromise. Black infants develop IVH at two times the rate of White infants despite overall improvements and decline in the rates of IVH within the past decade. This higher occurrence of IVH correlates with a higher rate of premature among infants born to Black mothers.[28] Segregation is known to increase racial and personal discrimination among minorities, increasing toxic stress in Black mothers, and negatively impacting maternal–infant care that includes increasing the risk of IVH.[29] Concern about racial disparity in the accuracy of pulse oximeters.[30,31] in the neonatal and pediatric population leading to unrecognized hypoxia among Black patients, potentially a driving factor in IVH outcomes. In addition, severe IVH continues to contribute to the rates of mortality from IVH and other complications such as cerebral palsy, which also show disparities by race.[32]

NECROTIZING ENTEROCOLITIS

In addition to developing IVH, Baby B also developed NEC. Complications from NEC are the leading cause of infant mortality for premature infants from 2 weeks to 2 months of life.[33] The exact etiology of NEC remains unknown, but several risk factors have been identified. The cascade of events culminating in an exaggerated inflammatory response and ultimate necrosis of portions or the entirety of the bowel is characteristic of this disease. This can be linked to the increased inflammatory response that the stress of racism causes in Black mothers, thereby increasing the risk of Black infants developing NEC.[10] This condition has approximately a 30% fatality rate and generally extends the NICU hospitalization one to 2 months if mortality from NEC does not ensue.[34] The use of breast milk or donor breast milk is known to reduce the risk of NEC in premature infants. However, breast milk use among Black infants is significantly lower.

BREASTFEEDING

Over the years, it has become evident that breast milk has many benefits for moms and infants. For moms, it increases bonding opportunities and decreases the risk of certain cancers. In addition to providing protective factors against NEC, breast milk is critical in improving infant brain development and reducing the development of chronic health conditions.[35] Although it is heavily promoted as the "gold standard" of nutrition for infants, there are significant differences in providing education and early lactation support to explain the benefits of breastfeeding or providing pumped breast milk among races.[15] Approximately 87% of infants born to White mothers have breastfeeding initiated, whereas only 74% of infants born to Black mothers have breastfeeding initiated. This gap only widens with time; only 48% of infants born to Black mothers are still receiving breast milk at 6 months, of life in contrast to 62% of infants born to White mothers.[3] This rate is even lower for infants requiring NICU care, as neonatal illness interferes with the establishment of breastfeeding and is instead reliant on their mothers to provide expressed breast milk, an additional logistic and financial barrier.[36]

Although efforts have begun to bridge this gap, there are still challenges in achieving breastfeeding parity between Black and White mothers.[37] This gap applies to breastfeeding extenders such as the use of donor breast milk, where Black mothers are less likely to consent.[10] Although the underlying factors remain under investigation, there is speculation that hospitals that serve higher populations of Black infants offer donor breast milk less often than those with a higher White population.[35]

Clinicians must be mindful of the cultural and historical context of breastfeeding for Black women. "Wet nursing," or the practice of breastfeeding a non-related child, was often imposed on Black slaves. As wet nursing could only be performed by women who had recently borne children of their own, it represented a unique form of exploitation practiced by at least one-fifth of slaveholding wives in the antebellum South.[38] This practice also meant that slaves were unable to adequately nurse their own infants due to reduced supply after feeding the White infants. Wet nursing along with hypersexualization of the bodies of Black women, and increased sexual violence helped to form negative connotations of breastfeeding in the Black community.[39] This cultural legacy was passed down for generations, with young mothers following the same practice of formula feeding as their mothers and grandmothers.

To bring about change, it is imperative that clinicians take extra time and consideration to provide additional education to Black mothers before and after the birth of their infants. Although feeding preference is a standard topic of conversation during visits by prenatal providers, failure to account for cultural differences when discussing the benefits or available resources for breastfeeding will inevitably lead to lower rates of breastfeeding. The lack of support from health care professionals has negatively impacted the initiation, continuation, and discharge of breastfeeding rates among Black mothers.[40]

Another important factor in breastfeeding rates is the support of employers and the community. Women with lower socioeconomic status often work jobs that are not breastfeeding-friendly. These jobs often do not have designated areas for pumping or give mothers the freedom to step away and pump whenever needed. These conditions often lead to a feeling of embarrassment and vulnerability in addition to unwanted negative attention from their managers or supervisors. This challenge especially plagues mothers of infants in the NICU. Prolonged hospitalization means that taking more away from work to be present at the hospital for family meetings, important procedures, and bonding with their infant[40] increases financial and job-related stress. The NICU imposes an additional logistic barrier on mothers; breast milk must be brought to the hospital on a regular basis. The lack of reliable transportation, lack of childcare for older children, or an overabundance of day-to-day responsibilities can contribute to mothers feeling overwhelmed and unable to pump consistently and provide breastmilk consistently.[36]

FAMILY EXPERIENCE

Reviewing the many medical complications Baby B developed during his hospitalization, we must remember that these were also experienced by the family of Baby B. A truly comprehensive approach integrates the entire family unit and should prioritize time, resources, and communication compared with that of Baby A. When this fails to occur, racism or discrimination must be considered as a root cause. Differences in the way marginalized groups are treated or perceive that they are treated remain a pernicious factor in health care and manifest in the form of disrespectful communication and dismissive behavior from health care providers. Clinicians should carefully examine how stereotyping and their own implicit bias shape their interactions and communication with minority families.[37] When ignored, further gaps in appropriate care develop, causing disparate care in the form of neglect, judgmental, or systemic barriers to care. This is especially noticed when the medical team is not mindful of the cultural and social norms that influence the decisions that families make about their infant's care.[10]

When families believe that they are being stereotyped, judged, or viewed negatively, there is the potential for less family interaction and visitation with their infants.[41] This becomes evident when rules are not enforced equally or resources are not distributed evenly among all the families. How an individual has had to maneuver through life when facing stereotypes in all areas of their lives can often have a direct impact on how they navigate interactions with health care professionals when faced with similar challenges.[19] Unfortunately, there is a correlation between chronic worry about racism and being treated unfairly and premature birth, with the highest rates among Black women with higher education and income brackets.[42] These women are often in positions where they must defend why they have a certain job or were given a particular opportunity. A lack of cultural competency and the inability to decode variations in language and nonverbal communication styles can lead to mothers being labeled as difficult or aggressive. Examples of this include speaking loudly or expressing themselves with their hands.[43] Other times, it is said that they are uninterested or have a flat affect because they do not ask questions or feel comfortable interacting with staff. This can cause chronic stress that impacts their physical health and causes constant cardio-vascular stress response.[44]

Qualitative research has captured the distress of Black families when their concerns are not heard or addressed when advocating for their infant.[19,41] They believed they were often talked down to and dismissed when they voiced concerns. One mother stated "...my fears and apprehensions were not acknowledged, and there wasn't any compassion there...I said, 'I don't know if you would do this to me if I were a married, White lady'... even if you have those feelings, deep in your heart, you shouldn't be bringing it outside" in a study by Glazer and colleagues. Sometimes, this was attributed to the tone of voice and demeanor of the health care professional, and sometimes, it was due to feeling as if the nurse or doctor was too busy to explain things in a manner they could understand. In another study by Witt and colleagues, one mother commented "I try to express to them that I want to be involved as much as I can, don't round without me ... But there were times where those requests were ignored ... It was more of if I didn't stay on top of it, I was going to get lost. I wasn't gonna be informed about what happened ... They just assumed that I was just a single Black mother." Communication styles play a significant role in the satisfaction of the families of infants in the NICU. Clear and candid communication, compassionate and supportive nurses, and nurses who genuinely wanted to help and educate families improved the family experience.[45]

There are many dissatisfiers for families during NICU hospitalization. For White families, the primary was the lack of continuity in nursing care. However, for Black families, it was reports of a lack of compassion, disrespectful communication, and inattention to their infant.[10] In hospitals with high Black patient populations, nurses missed almost 50% more nursing care activities compared with hospitals that serve a lower proportion of Black patients. Most often, these activities included teaching families and providing comfort to the infants and their families. A higher ratio of public payors (e.g., Medicaid and Medicare) versus private payors can lead to an increased financial burden for the hospital and implementation of cost reduction programs, including a reduction in payroll. When staffing challenges happen, it results in higher nurse-to-patient ratios, shifting the labor focus to compulsory medical duties, leaving less time to interact with families and teach them how to care for their infants.[46]

There is increasing evidence that Black patients have better outcomes, including reduced mortality when cared for by Black providers.[47] In qualitative analysis, the family experience was impacted when Black mothers encountered Black staff; they felt more comfortable expressing concerns and that their message was heard. This was especially true when those concerns involved cultural differences such as skin and hair care. They also felt that Black nurses were more likely to advocate for their infants and keep them updated on important information. Black nurses were also more likely to take extra time to assist with breastfeeding concerns and teach families how to care for their infants.[19]

Unfortunately, the health care workforce lacks adequate representation with 6.7% of nurses[48] and 5.0% of physicians[49] identifying as Black, despite making up 13.6% of the total US population. Major stakeholders in the health care arena have agreed that diversifying the workforce should be a priority. This is something that must start at the nursing and medical school level with intentional recruitment and retention of underrepresented minority groups. Diversification of leadership and administrators to better resemble the patient population will also lead to having a better diverse health system that can aid in having a better family experience for Black families.[48]

RECOMMENDATIONS

As is frequently the case in neonatology, more research is needed to truly understand the ramifications of racism on this vulnerable population.[50] The first step health care professionals must take to begin the process of mitigating health disparities is to acknowledge the problem and look internally to recognize any personal bias and understand that past experiences and interactions shape future interactions.[51] It is important to understand cultural differences as well as the individual nature of each patient's family. Resources that include follow-up appointments, nursing visits, and community programs should also be used according to what the families determine their needs are instead of solely being determined by hospital staff without incorporating the main social determinant of health into the equation. Consideration for schedules, lifestyles, and means should be discussed with family members when planning care for the infant. Another important factor that must be taken into consideration is that of workplace diversity. Representation matters and organizations should take an internal look at why there are so few minorities in professional and leadership positions and the impact that has on the patients and the families we care for.

SUMMARY

Racism is an embedded part of the history of the United States. Slavery was legal in North America for 246 years and dramatically altered the reproductive health of Black women and the well-being of their children. After the end of the Civil War, legal discrimination through segregation and Jim Crow policies remained enforced through political and legal power structures. Even after the Civil Rights era of the 1960s, the impact of hundreds of years of racism continues to be felt through deeply embedded structural racism.

Health care is no exception to this legacy, through explicitly racist experiments such as the Tuskegee Study of Untreated Syphilis, continued teaching of insidious and disproven theories of intellectual inferiority or higher pain tolerances,[52] or abuses of power such as the creation of the HeLa immortal cell line. These cells were taken from Henrietta Lacks, a Black woman being treated for an extremely aggressive cervical cancer, without her consent and are still widely used today in research.[53] These deceptive practices have led to generations of mistrust and suspicion of the healthcare system for Black families, and it is imperative that health care professionals keep this in mind when trying to establish a trusting relationship.

To move forward, health care professionals must acknowledge the past and commit to working together to eliminate health disparities. Access to health care in areas that were previously redlined, increased resources to hospitals that take care of high Black populations, improving local access to prenatal care, and more representative staffing would help to improve maternal health through a reduction in premature birth. For those infants still born prematurely, care focused on reducing disparities will continue to lower the rates of neonatal morbidities and mortality, increase breastfeeding rates, and promote healthy family experiences.

CLINICS CARE POINTS

- Premature birth rates are higher in the United States than any other upper income country and are associated with a high infant mortality rate, with Black infants being born prematurely at two times the rate of white infants.

- Health care professionals must keep in mind the lived experiences of generations of Black families that reinforce the suspicion and mistrust of the healthcare system when trying to establish a trusting relationship with Black families.
- Acknowledge the problem of health disparities and begin the process of mitigating them prior to birth.
- Can we commit to working together collaboratively with families to eliminate health disparities?

DISCLOSURE

The authors have nothing to disclose.

REFERENCES

1. Oliveira KA de, Araújo EM de, Oliveira KA de, et al. Association between race/skin color and premature birth: a systematic review with meta-analysis. Rev Saude Publica 2018;52:26.
2. Morales LS, Staiger D, Horbar JD, et al. Mortality among very low-birthweight infants in hospitals serving minority populations. Am J Public Health 2005;95(12):2206–12.
3. Reports for United States. March of Dimes | PeriStats https://www.marchofdimes.org/peristats/reports/united-states. Accessed June 28, 2023.
4. Johnson JD, Green CA, Vladutiu CJ, et al. Racial disparities in prematurity persist among women of high socioeconomic status. Am J Obstet Gynecol MFM 2020;2(3):100104.
5. da Silva PHA, Aiquoc KM, da Silva Nunes AD, et al. Prevalence of access to prenatal care in the first trimester of pregnancy among black women compared to other races/Ethnicities: a systematic review and meta-analysis. Public Health Rev 2022;43:1604400.
6. Barfield WD. Public health implications of very preterm birth. Clin Perinatol 2018;45(3):565–77.
7. Elias A, Paradies Y. The costs of institutional racism and its Ethical implications for healthcare. J Bioethical Inq 2021;18(1):45–58.
8. What is structural racism? American Medical Association. Published November 9, 2021. Accessed June 28, 2023. https://www.ama-assn.org/delivering-care/health-equity/what-structural-racism.
9. Racism and Health. Centers for Disease Control and Prevention. Published November 24, 2021. Accessed June 28, 2023. https://www.cdc.gov/minorityhealth/racism-disparities/index.html.
10. Sigurdson K, Mitchell B, Liu J, et al. Racial/ethnic disparities in neonatal intensive care: a systematic review. Pediatrics 2019;144(2):e20183114.
11. Bailey ZD, Feldman JM, Bassett MT. How structural racism works — racist policies as a root cause of U.S. Racial health inequities. In: Malina D, editor. N Engl J Med 2021;384(8):768–73.
12. Locke DH, Hall B, Grove JM, et al. Residential housing segregation and urban tree canopy in 37 US Cities. Npj Urban Sustain 2021;1(1):15.
13. Yeokwang An, Bostic RW, Jakabovics A, Orlando AW, Rodnyansky S. Small and Medium Multifamily Housing Units: Affordability, Distribution, and Trends. Published online 2017. doi:10.13140/RG.2.2.18740.14722.

14. An B, Orlando AW, Rodnyansky S. The physical legacy of racism: how redlining cemented the modern built environment. SSRN Electron J 2019. https://doi.org/10.2139/ssrn.3500612.

15. Ravi D, Iacob A, Profit J. Unequal care: racial/ethnic disparities in neonatal intensive care delivery. Semin Perinatol 2021;45(4):151411.

16. Liu J, Sakarovitch C, Sigurdson K, et al. Disparities in health care–associated infections in the NICU. Am J Perinatol 2020;37(02):166–73.

17. Montoya-Williams D, Fraiman YS, Peña MM, et al. Antiracism in the field of Neonatology: a Foundation and concrete approaches. NeoReviews 2022; 23(1):e1–12.

18. Huang SJ, Sehgal NJ. Association of historic redlining and present-day health in Baltimore. In: Liu SY, editor. PLoS One 2022;17(1):e0261028. https://doi.org/10.1371/journal.pone.0261028.

19. Witt RE, Malcolm M, Colvin BN, et al. Racism and quality of neonatal intensive care: voices of black mothers. Pediatrics 2022;150(3). e2022056971.

20. Lorch SA, Rogowski J, Profit J, et al. Access to risk-appropriate hospital care and disparities in neonatal outcomes in racial/ethnic groups and rural–urban populations. Semin Perinatol 2021;45(4):151409.

21. Travers CP, Carlo WA, McDonald SA, et al. Racial/ethnic disparities among extremely preterm infants in the United States from 2002 to 2016. JAMA Netw Open 2020;3(6):e206757.

22. Wallace M, Crear-Perry J, Richardson L, et al. Separate and unequal: structural racism and infant mortality in the US. Health Place 2017;45:140–4.

23. Getting Hyperlocal to Improve Outcomes & Achieve Racial Equity in Maternal Health: The US Maternal Vulnerability Index — Surgo Ventures https://surgoventures.org/resource-library/getting-hyperlocal-to-improve-outcomes-achieve-racial-equity-in-maternal-health-the-us-mvi. Accessed June 28, 2023.

24. Riddell CA, Harper S, Kaufman JS. Trends in differences in US mortality rates between black and white infants. JAMA Pediatr 2017;171(9):911.

25. Wallace ME, Mendola P, Kim SS, et al. Racial/ethnic differences in preterm perinatal outcomes. Am J Obstet Gynecol 2017;216(3):306.e1–12.

26. Gleibner M, Jorch G, Avenarius S. Risk factors for intraventricular hemorrhage in a birth cohort of 3721 premature infants. J Perinat Med 2000;28(2).

27. Vesoulis ZA, Bank RL, Lake D, et al. Early hypoxemia burden is strongly associated with severe intracranial hemorrhage in preterm infants. J Perinatol Off J Calif Perinat Assoc 2019;39(1):48–53.

28. Qureshi AI, Adil MM, Shafizadeh N, et al. A 2-fold higher rate of intraventricular hemorrhage–related mortality in African American neonates and infants: clinical article. J Neurosurg Pediatr 2013;12(1):49–53.

29. Murosko D, Passerella M, Lorch S. Racial segregation and intraventricular hemorrhage in preterm infants. Pediatrics 2020;145(6). e20191508.

30. Foglia EE, Whyte RK, Chaudhary A, et al. The effect of skin pigmentation on the accuracy of pulse oximetry in infants with hypoxemia. J Pediatr 2017;182:375–7.e2.

31. Vesoulis Z, Tims A, Lodhi H, et al. Racial discrepancy in pulse oximeter accuracy in preterm infants. J Perinatol Off J Calif Perinat Assoc 2022;42(1):79–85.

32. Wu YW, Xing G, Fuentes-Afflick E, et al. Racial, ethnic, and socioeconomic disparities in the prevalence of cerebral palsy. Pediatrics 2011;127(3):e674–81.

33. Wolf MF, Rose AT, Goel R, et al. Trends and racial and geographic differences in infant mortality in the United States due to necrotizing enterocolitis, 1999 to 2020. JAMA Netw Open 2023;6(3):e231511.
34. Lake ET, Staiger D, Horbar J, et al. Disparities in perinatal quality outcomes for very low birth weight infants in neonatal intensive care. Health Serv Res 2015; 50(2):374–97.
35. Parker MG, Gupta M, Melvin P, et al. Racial and ethnic disparities in the Use of Mother's milk feeding for very low birth weight infants in Massachusetts. J Pediatr 2019;204:134–41.e1.
36. Riley B, Schoeny M, Rogers L, et al. Barriers to Human milk feeding at discharge of very low–Birthweight infants: evaluation of neighborhood structural factors. Breastfeed Med 2016;11(7):335–42.
37. Ravi D, Profit J. Disparities in neonatal intensive care: causes, consequences and charting the path forward. Semin Perinatol 2021;45(4):151406.
38. West E, Knight RJ. Mothers' milk: slavery, wet-nursing, and black and white women in the antebellum South. J South Hist 2017;83(1):37–68.
39. Petit M, Smart DA, Sattler V, et al. Examination of factors that contribute to breast-feeding disparities and Inequities for black women in the US. J Nutr Educ Behav 2021;53(11):977–86.
40. Spencer B, Wambach K, Domain EW. African American Women's breastfeeding experiences: cultural, personal, and political voices. Qual Health Res 2015;25(7): 974–87.
41. Glazer KB, Sofaer S, Balbierz A, et al. Perinatal care experiences among racially and ethnically diverse mothers whose infants required a NICU stay. J Perinatol 2021;41(3):413–21.
42. Braveman P, Heck K, Egerter S, et al. Worry about racial discrimination: a missing piece of the puzzle of Black-White disparities in preterm birth? Ryckman KK. PLoS One 2017;12(10):e0186151.
43. Lewis JA, Mendenhall R, Harwood SA, et al. "Ain't I a woman?": perceived Gendered racial microaggressions experienced by black women. Couns Psychol 2016;44(5):758–80.
44. Sawyer PJ, Major B, Casad BJ, et al. Discrimination and the stress response: psy-chological and physiological consequences of anticipating prejudice in inter-ethnic interactions. Am J Public Health 2012;102(5):1020–6.
45. Martin AE, D'Agostino JA, Passarella M, et al. Racial differences in parental satis-faction with neonatal intensive care unit nursing care. J Perinatol 2016;36(11): 1001–7.
46. Lake ET, Staiger D, Edwards EM, et al. Nursing care disparities in neonatal inten-sive care units. Health Serv Res 2018;53:3007–26.
47. Snyder JE, Upton RD, Hassett TC, et al. Black representation in the primary care physician workforce and its association with population life expectancy and mor-tality rates in the US. JAMA Netw Open 2023;6(4):e236687.
48. Enhancing Diversity in the Nursing Workforce https://www.aacnnursing.org/news-data/fact-sheets/enhancing-diversity-in-the-nursing-workforce. Accessed June 29, 2023.
49. Figure 18. Percentage of all active physicians by race/ethnicity, 2018. AAMC https://www.aamc.org/data-reports/workforce/data/figure-18-percentage-all-active-physicians-race/ethnicity-2018. Accessed June 29, 2023.
50. Parker MG, Hwang SS. Quality improvement approaches to reduce racial/ ethnic disparities in the neonatal intensive care unit. Semin Perinatol 2021; 45(4):151412.

51. Horbar JD, Edwards EM, Greenberg LT, et al. Racial segregation and inequality in the neonatal intensive care Unit for very low-birth-weight and very preterm infants. JAMA Pediatr 2019;173(5):455.
52. Hardeman RR, Medina EM, Kozhimannil KB. Structural racism and supporting black lives — the role of health professionals. N Engl J Med 2016;375(22): 2113–5.
53. Beskow LM. Lessons from HeLa Cells: The Ethics and Policy of Biospecimens. Annu Rev Genomics Hum Genet 2016;17:395–417.

Care from Birth to Discharge of Infants Born at 22 to 23 Weeks' Gestation

John M. Dagle, MD, PhD[a,b,*], Stephen K. Hunter, MD, PhD[c],
Tarah T. Colaizy, MD, MPH[a,b], Steve J. McElroy, MD[d],
Heidi M. Harmon, MD[a,b], Patrick J. McNamara, MD, MSc[a,b,e],
Jonathan M. Klein, MD[a,b]

KEYWORDS

- Extreme prematurity • Outcomes • Precision

KEY POINTS

- Importance of care design: Proper care for infants born at 22 weeks' gestation is crucial for best results.
- Consistency is key: Care protocols should be well-structured and consistent, avoiding randomness.
- University of Iowa example: The University of Iowa Stead Family Children's Hospital Neonatal Intensive Care Unit shares its approach for babies born at 22 weeks' gestation.
- Comprehensive care plan: This standardized plan covers prenatal, neurologic, nutritional, gastrointestinal, and skin care.
- Focused review: Respiratory and cardiopulmonary care is briefly discussed, building upon previously published strategies and considering the unique anatomy and physiology of these infants.

INTRODUCTION

Survival for extremely preterm infants has improved dramatically over the past 20 years.[1] The advances responsible for improved survival are multifactorial and relate

All authors reviewed and provided feedback on the final version of the manuscript.
Sources of Financial Assistance: None.
[a] Division of Neonatology, Department of Pediatrics, University of Iowa, Iowa City, IA, USA;
[b] University of Iowa Stead Family Children's Hospital, Iowa City, IA, USA; [c] Department of Obstetrics & Gynecology, University of Iowa, Iowa City, IA, USA; [d] Division of Neonatology, Department of Pediatrics, University of California, Davis, Sacramento, CA, USA; [e] Department of Internal Medicine, University of Iowa, Iowa City, IA, USA
* Corresponding author. Division of Neonatology, Department of Pediatrics, University of Iowa, Iowa City, IA.
E-mail address: john-dagle@uiowa.edu

to increased appreciation of organ vulnerability, enhanced diagnostic precision, and improved therapeutic options. In addition to standardizing the approach to clinical care and longitudinal monitoring of physiologic stability and nutritional health, the establishment of cohesive teams which function within a uniform unit culture is paramount. A proactive approach must begin before birth and continues throughout the hospitalization to minimize variability in how the medical and nursing teams care for infants born below 24 weeks' gestation. Integral to the performance of the team is acceptance of a mutually agreed philosophic approach and ongoing education within an immersive learning environment. There must also be an understanding and acceptance that mortality may be higher in this group as we continue to optimize care plans. Unfortunately, the advances that underlie enhanced survival do not always guarantee avoidance of adverse long-term outcomes. In addition, life-saving treatments may have potential, unintended negative biological effects on subsequent organ development. Despite these caveats, employing standardized therapies based on the biology of our youngest patients has resulted in improved survival with good quality of life.

In this report, we highlight the developmental vulnerability of immature organ systems and review common diseases of infants born at the limits of viability. Specifically, we outline the principles of the approach to resuscitation, thermoregulation, fluid balance and nutrition, ventilation assistance, hemodynamic care, and neuroprotective strategies that constitute routine care in our quaternary neonatal intensive care unit (NICU). The University of Iowa NICU is a quaternary referral center with 87 beds, which includes a 12-bed neonatal critical care unit where extremely preterm infants are initially managed. Based on the link between extreme prematurity, abnormal organ development, and long-term risk of adverse outcomes, we propose the need for routine, standardized frameworks for the assessment and monitoring of physiologic phenotypes in premature infants.

APPROACH TO THE CARE OF MOTHERS WHO DELIVER AT 22 WEEKS

Successful outcomes of extremely premature infants do not begin in the NICU, nor do they rely solely on neonatal interventions. The path to achieving outstanding outcomes begins before birth and involves collaboration and coordination of practices developed by maternal-fetal-medicine (MFM) physicians with those developed by neonatologists. There must be mutual trust and effective communication between MFM physicians and neonatologists as part of the shared decision-making process. It is important to recognize that the protocols described below may be outside the recommendations of national organizations (eg, American Congress of Obstetricians and Gynecologists) and are based on the institutional outcomes at Iowa and guided by an absolute commitment to the health and well-being of the mother first and foremost. From an obstetric perspective, the life and well-being of the mother always take precedence over that of her extremely preterm fetus; nevertheless, MFM physicians always do their best to deliver the healthiest possible infant. At our institution, each patient at risk of delivering an extremely premature infant has a discussion with a neonatologist prior to delivery (if possible) to discuss the impact of intensive care support at 22 weeks' gestational age (GA). The MFM physician also discusses in detail, the risks and benefits of all therapies, including the competing impact of the administration of antenatal steroids at $21^{5/7}$ and $21^{6/7}$ weeks to maternal versus fetal health. If a mother is known to have a significant risk for extreme premature delivery, that is, preterm prolonged rupture of membranes before 22 weeks, admission to our institution at $21^{5/7}$ weeks is offered to begin the administration of antenatal steroids, if she desires active resuscitation at 22 weeks. Importantly, the decision to give antenatal corticosteroids is separate from the decision to intervene with cesarean section. Antenatal magnesium sulfate is administered for neuroprotection of the immature brain.

The delivery method is also discussed extensively with the mother. As there is little information regarding any benefit of cesarean over vaginal delivery at GAs less than 24 weeks, and knowing the additive risks to the mother, a threshold of greater than or equal to 24 weeks is generally used for routinely offering cesarean delivery, regardless of fetal tolerance to the labor process or presentation of the fetus (vertex or breech). In individualized situations, cesarean delivery may be offered during the 22nd and 23rd weeks of gestation. It is, however, important to highlight the increased likelihood of a classical cesarean section at these GAs, which will affect all future pregnancies. The patient is also informed that, regardless of the type of cesarean section (classical vs low transverse), the risk for life-threatening uterine rupture or morbidly adherent placenta syndrome is increased in future pregnancies. Finally, fetal monitoring during labor at extremely low GA is discussed, which again relies heavily on the desires of the parents. Some families may choose not to have fetal monitoring before 23 weeks as a cesarean section may not be offered even in the event of fetal intolerance to labor.

APPROACH TO THE IMMATURE BRAIN

Supporting optimal neuromaturation and development focuses on 3 key elements: intraventricular hemorrhage (IVH) prevention, support of appropriate brain growth with reduction of white matter injury, and facilitation of parental engagement and bonding. A specialized neurocritical care team is available to provide guidance to this high-risk population. Because of the increased risk of severe IVH in extremely preterm infants, efforts in the perinatal period and early postnatal period are strongly focused on prevention of IVH. Obstetric practices to reduce the risk of IVH include maternal transport prior to delivery, universal antenatal steroids administration combined with the use of magnesium (as a tocolytic to allow for steroid completion and for neuroprotection), and delayed cord clamping. Resuscitation efforts that also support a neuroprotective strategy include careful handling, maintenance of thermoregulation, and restricting intubation to experienced providers.

Postnatal IVH prevention strategies focus on reducing fluctuations in cerebral blood flow through precision in fluid management, hemodynamic intervention, and ventilation strategies. Frequent laboratory assessment (every 2–3 hours) in the transitional period allows for rapid correction of physiologic factors that may contribute to IVH. By avoiding hypercapnia or hypocapnia, fluctuations of cerebral blood flow may be avoided. Glucose is also closely monitored and kept within a range of 50 to 150 mg/dL. We transfuse for hemoglobin less than 11.5 g/dL to avoid early anemia, with packed red blood cells coming from a single donor to reduce infection risk. A single oral dose of vitamin E, an antioxidant, is provided shortly after birth to reduce IVH risk.[2] Nursing protocols recommend the avoidance of aggressive suctioning or noxious stimuli that induce abrupt elevations in blood pressure. In addition, clinical examinations are deferred to every 4-hour cluster cares to preserve sleep and reduce infant agitation. During cares, lighting is dim, eyes are shielded, and noise is minimized. During the first 2 postnatal weeks positioning is supine with head in midline and flexion of arms, legs, and shoulders within nested boundaries. Parents are encouraged to interact by gentle static touch during this period. Routine neuromonitoring (near-infrared spectroscopy, electroencephalography) is currently restricted to the highest risk patients due to skin integrity issues and reducing unnecessary handling in the first postnatal week. A limited head ultrasound is completed by hemodynamic faculty as part of the first targeted neonatal echocardiography (TnECHO) assessment, which is clustered with other cares between 12 and 18 hours of life. A formal head ultrasound is deferred until days 5 to 7 unless there is evidence of brain injury on the initial screen or cerebral dysfunction is suggested by clinical symptoms.

Brain development is actively supported throughout the hospitalization. A preventative approach to inflammatory conditions (e.g., necrotizing enterocolitis [NEC], spontaneous intestinal perforation [SIP], and late onset- sepsis), which compromise white matter injury and dysmaturation, is used. The approach to respiratory management prioritizes the maintenance of stable oxygen and CO_2 homeostasis, rather than focusing on early extubation. Empiric caffeine is provided within the first 24 hours with liberal use of additional caffeine doses to address persistent or recurrent apnea. Unintended extubation is rare and elective extubation is deferred until success is considered likely (often around a weight approaching 900 g). Severe apnea spells following extubation are managed by use of noninvasive neurally adjusted ventilatory assist (NAVA). As part of a neuroprotective strategy, we avoid routine sedatives and opiates in intubated preterm infants, as these agents have negative effects on brain maturation, and high-frequency jet ventilation (HFJV) is generally well tolerated in this population. If phenobarbital is needed for seizures related to IVH, attempts are made to wean this medication as soon as appropriate. Optimal nutrition and strong support of maternal breast milk are emphasized within the unit to facilitate improved neurodevelopmental outcomes, as is the use of probiotics. Involvement of physical therapy, occupation therapy, and child life specialists is important for both development of the premature infant and for family education. The central role of family is recognized as one of the largest contributors to infant outcomes. Parents are welcome in the NICU and are encouraged to be present during rounds and participate in daily infant care. Parent holding and kangaroo care are encouraged after 2 weeks of age. Social workers and psychologists provide screening for postpartum depression and can provide services at the bedside.

APPROACH TO FLUID AND NUTRITIONAL MANAGEMENT

Central umbilical venous (UVC) and arterial catheters (UAC) are attempted, within 60 minutes of birth, in all infants born at 22 weeks' GA; specifically, 3.5 Fr catheters are used with the UVC (double lumen) and UAC (single lumen) placed at ~6 cm and ~10, respectively. The umbilical lines are kept in place for as long as they are needed, with no preset limit on the duration of use. Inadequate access for these critically ill infants can become a significant issue limiting optimal care, especially with frequent lab studies, up to every 3 hours. Infants in this age group are managed on radiant warmers for the first few weeks after birth to allow continuous visualization and immediate, unhindered access. In addition, earlier skin keratinization seen with this decreased humidity may protect against infection.[3] This approach results in increased insensible fluid losses compared with care in incubators requiring higher fluid intake in the first 1 to 2 weeks of life. Fluids are initiated at 150 to 200 mL/kg/ day and titrated to maintain stable water homeostasis. Sterile water with sodium acetate (approximately 40 meq/L) is infused at 1.5 mL/h through the UAC. Total parental nutrition (TPN) solution (with minimal sodium containing 7.5% dextrose and 5% amino acids) is started through the UVC at 30 to 50 mL/kg/d to provide 1.5 to 2 g/kg/d of protein immediately after birth. An additional 2.5% to 5% dextrose/water carrier fluid is infused through the UVC and is adjusted to maintain water, sodium, and glucose homeostasis. The goal is to consistently provide the ordered TPN, if possible, to ensure protein for growth. If hyperglycemia becomes an issue, the glucose infusion rate (GIR) is reduced. It must be remembered that the goal of a glucose infusion is to ensure euglycemia and that maintaining an arbitrarily elevated GIR in the face of hyperglycemia should be avoided. Intravenous insulin is rarely used unless blood glucose remains greater than 200 mg/dL with a GIR of less than 2 mg/kg/min. Heparin is generally included in only one fluid in each catheter (0.25 U/mL) to keep the daily heparin dose at less than 75 U/kg/d. Blood glucose and electrolytes are monitored every 3 hours until stable, and fluid volume is adjusted based on daily weights, urine output, serum and/or urine sodium, or TnECHO evidence of hydration deficits. The smallest and most immature infants may require greater than 200 mL/kg/d for several days to maintain intravascular volume. Custom TPN with lipid infusion is administered as soon as feasible (generally within 24 hours), with a protein intake of 3 to 3.5 g/kg/d and an initial lipid dose of 1 g/kg/d (intralipid), which is increased to a final target dose of 2 g/kg/d on postnatal day 2 to 3. Daily TPN protein infusion is maintained at 3.5 to 4 g/kg/d until the TPN rate is weaned to 80 mL/kg/d, the point that this protein administration cannot be achieved with a 5% amino acid solution.

Enteral nutrition is started within 24 hours of birth using unfortified human milk. Ideally, maternal colostrum is used; however, if this is not available, pasteurized donor milk from the Mother's Milk Bank of Iowa is used. Infant formula is generally not fed to infants born at 22 weeks' gestation until 34 to 36 weeks postmenstrual age (when maternal discharge preferences are initiated). Feedings are started at a low volume (5–10 mL/kg/day divided every 8–12 hours) and increased daily or every other day by 10 mL/kg/day for the first 7 to 10 days if the infant is tolerating the feed and stooling daily. The rate of augmentation of feeds is typically reduced in patients with a hemodynamically significant patent ductus arteriosus (PDA), severe intrauterine growth restriction, or in patients with evidence of a hypoxic-ischemic event. After 7 to 10 days, daily enteral volume is increased by 15 to 20 mL/kg/d to achieve a goal intake of at least 150 mL/kg/d. Feedings are infused every 3 to 4 hours, on a pump over 60 minutes until infants are a month old. Bovine human milk fortifier is added when an infant is receiving 25 mL of human milk per day and greater than 7 days, regardless of infant weight, if feedings are well tolerated. This helps to ensure the desired intake of calcium, phosphorous and protein (which normally accrues later in gestation), in addition to additional calories.

Replacement sodium is almost universally needed to enhance growth and is guided by urinary sodium excretion, which can be used to measure total body sodium in this population.[4] Supplementation, in the first 2 months, is initially provided in TPN but subsequently via the enteral route. The approach to fluid and electrolyte homeostasis requires frequent longitudinal monitoring that enables a high degree of precision in diagnosis and care. See **Table 1** for a summary of specific aspects of nutritional management.

APPROACH TO THE IMMATURE RESPIRATORY SYSTEM

A first-intention high-frequency approach is our standard of care for extremely preterm infants with respiratory distress syndrome.[5] Recognizing that infants at 22 weeks' GA have limited alveolar development, it is critically important to reduce the risk of volutrauma as the lungs are susceptible to acquiring pulmonary interstitial emphysema. Infants are universally intubated in the delivery room, often with a size 2.0 mm (93% of 22 week GA) internal diameter endotracheal tubes.[6] We recently published a comprehensive report on respiratory management in this vulnerable population.[7]

The initial HFJV strategy focuses on avoiding mechanical injury from air-trapping and air leaks. The initial jet rate is set at 300 breaths per minute, with the I-time set

Table 1 Aspects of nutritional management used at the University of Iowa	
Strategy	**Rationale**
Use of radiant warmers	Allows for continuous observation and immediate access. This also leads to increased fluid intake, which requires frequent monitoring and frequent fluid adjustments. This strategy does allow for full TPN administration immediately from birth and reduces the protein deficit experienced by many extremely preterm infants.
Standardized feeding protocols based on slow feeding advancement	Allows for slower gastrointestinal adaptation to enteral feedings, which impacts our low NEC rates. Prolonged TPN administration enables maximization of protein intake to further decrease protein deficit. This may, however, lead to a longer central line exposure time.
Prolonged use of donor breast milk	As the NEC risk window extends to 34 wk PMA, exclusive use of human milk and probiotics throughout this period is the standard.
Early institution of human milk fortification	Goal is to further enhance nutritional health and optimize organ development/rehabilitation. Careful attention to protein and energy intake to avoid postnatal growth failure.
Sodium surveillance and aggressive supplementation	Strategy used to optimize growth.

at 20 milliseconds, which provides an inspiratory: expiratory (I:E) ratio of 1:9. An initial positive end-expiratory pressure of 5 cm is chosen to avoid hyperinflation leading to impaired venous return with a potential impact on cerebral blood flow. The initial peak inspiratory pressure (PIP) is usually started at 22 to 24 cm and adjusted as needed until visible but not excessive jet vibrations of the chest wall are achieved. PIPs are subsequently adjusted to maintain tight control of Pco_2 values. Background intermittent mandatory ventilation breaths are not initially started on HFJV.

Early extubation is avoided in this fragile population due to increased mortality and morbidity associated with a failed attempt.[8] Infants are extubated to noninvasive ventilation using NAVA which uses the electrical activity generated by the diaphragm during its activation to synchronize and proportionally assist each spontaneous patient breath.

APPROACH TO THE IMMATURE CARDIOVASCULAR SYSTEM

Early identification of pathology is particularly essential for 22 week infants as many cardiopulmonary diseases have substantial overlap in clinical phenotype, and these neonates have limited capability to adapt to even subtle derangements in physiology. Clinical evaluation of hypotension is challenging in this patient population as normative data have not been established. An approach using systolic (presumed low cardiac output) versus diastolic (presumed systemic vasodilation) predominant patterns may be helpful in delineating the cause of hypotension and can be used to adjudicate the most appropriate first-line therapy. First-line therapies for low systolic arterial pressure (or heart dysfunction) include intravenous dobutamine or low-dose epinephrine, and therapy for low diastolic pressure is intravenous norepinephrine. In patients with acute pulmonary hypertension intravenous vasopressin is typically chosen due to its more favorable effects on the pulmonary vascular bed. Because of the increased vulnerability of the immature myocardium to changes in loading conditions, a disease-based approach to treatment selection, rather than focusing on arbitrary symptom-based thresholds, is considered desirable.[9] Early screening (<24 hours) with echocardiography allows earlier identification of abnormal disease state, enhanced phenotypic characterization, and a more precise approach to treatment selection. Specific details of this approach are published elsewhere.[7] Intravenous acetaminophen is the first-line treatment of patients with evidence of a hemodynamically significant PDA. Low-dose inhaled nitric oxide (5–10 ppm) is used for patients with hypoxemic respiratory failure and echocardiography evidence of pulmonary hypertension to mitigate major swings in transductal, and hence cerebral, blood flow. Early hemodynamics screening and a targeted approach to cardiovascular intervention were associated with a 50% reduction in the composite of death or grade III/IV IVH.[10] Early identification and treatment of a hemodynamically significant PDA was also found to decrease the risk of severe bronchopulmonary dysplasia and necrotizing enterocolitis.

APPROACH TO THE IMMATURE GASTROINTESTINAL TRACT

Consideration of the intestinal tract is essential when caring for infants at 22 weeks. The massive surface of the intestine must protect the host from the harsh acidic environment of the stomach, the digestive enzymes produced by the pancreas, and the bacteria that live (for the most part, symbiotically) in the intestinal tract and outnumber the cells in our bodies.[11,12] The intestine of the preterm infant is in constant developmental flux, changing with each week of GA.[13] By 8 to 12 weeks of gestation, villi, microvilli, and crypt structures begin to form, and by the end of the first trimester most major epithelial cell types, including absorptive enterocytes and secretory cells (Paneth cells, goblet cells, and enteroendocrine cells), have appeared.[14] However, by 22 to 24 weeks GA, fetuses do not yet consistently secrete digestive enzymes, do not have a normal gastric emptying or intestinal motility, and are not yet producing term-equivalent levels of the antimicrobial peptides that help to prevent pathogen invasion of the intestine.[13–17]

The intestinal tract of infants at 22 weeks is particularly susceptible to 3 major diseases, NEC, spontaneous focal intestinal perforation (often abbreviated SIP, IP, or FIP), and intestinal perforation resulting from inspissated meconium. The incidence of NEC in infants with birth weight less than 1000 g varies widely among developed countries, ranging from 5% to 22%,[18] and in the United States is around 7%.[19] Risk factors associated with the development of NEC in the preterm infant include degree of prematurity, low birth weight, formula feeding, intestinal ischemia, prolonged antibiotic use, and anemia.[20–24] The incidence of SIP has been reported to be 1% in infants born at 32 weeks of gestation or less and 2.3% in infants born at 28 weeks of gestation or less.[25] Importantly, over the past 10 years, the rate of NEC in 22 and 23-week infants cared for at Iowa is 6.2% (compared with 2.6% in infants born at 24–26 weeks), and our rate of SIP is 5%, suggesting that these profoundly preterm infants have an increased susceptibility to these disease processes. Neither disease has a reliable biomarker, so both conditions require careful daily monitoring of feeding tolerance. The infants need to be assessed for signs of abdominal pathology, such as distention or development of visible "blue spots" on the bowel wall that can represent meconium in the peritoneal cavity. They may present with a gasless abdomen following intestinal perforation; so, while assessing with abdominal radiography is critical, the utilization of abdominal ultrasound has greatly improved our diagnostic ability. Inspissated meconium has been appreciated more frequently with decreasing GA, resulting in the development of a standardized approach to this condition, described below.

Box 1
Approaches to skin care at the University of Iowa

- Skin care is vital—stratum corneum may be as thin as a few cells thick. Extremely low birth weight infants may need as many as 8 weeks for the stratum corneum to provide an effective barrier.
- Minimal use of skin adhesives to prevent separation between the dermis and epidermis.
- Use nonadhesive Velcro wrap oximeter cuff for all infants less than 26 weeks for the first 2 weeks of life.
- Change oximeter probe and temperature probe site every 8 hours.
- Use micro-electrocardiogram leads. May place patches of Mepitel One (Mölnlycke Health Care, Peachtree Corners, GA, USA) under ECG leads to prevent excoriation and breakdown.
- Chemicals may damage or be absorbed through the skin and should be avoided. Wipe off alcohol, betadine, etc. with sterile water if they must be used.
- Sween 24 Cream (Coloplast, Minneapolis, MN, USA) is recommended for daily use but can be applied up to every 8 hours as needed for dry skin.
- Triad cream can be used on wounds as needed for infants greater than 25 weeks' gestation.
- Keep perineal area protected by maintenance of barrier paste such as Criticaid Clear or Criticaid Paste (Coloplast, Minneapolis, MN, USA).
- Minimize adhesive tape use. Use adhesive remover sparingly with removal of tapes.
- Use soft disposable cloths with water to clean diaper area. Do not use diaper wipes for infants less than 28 weeks' gestation and 2 weeks of age. Water wipes may be considered after 2 weeks' PMA.
- Cover wounds and cracks on skin with Mepitel dressing. May apply Sween 24 over Mepitel One. Replace dressings when no longer adhering to skin.
- Do not bathe until greater than 2 weeks of age. Use only water until 32 weeks' gestation.
- Assess skin for pressure ulcer development daily and as needed.
- Assess skin at least every 12 hours using a standard scoring system.

Four quality improvement practices have been instituted at our program to help prevent intestinal complications in this cohort. As highlighted earlier, feeds are initiated early but advanced slowly. Although this increases the time to full feeds, it has not adversely impacted clinical outcomes.[1] The second is a heavy reliance on human milk-preferably fresh maternal milk and, when not available, donor milk. The third is the routine use of glycerin suppositories (which are cut to size) if these infants do not stool for more than 48 hours. The confluence of small intestinal diameter with impaired peristalsis and relative dehydration contributes to impaired intestinal function and difficulty moving meconium. If glycerin suppositories are ineffective, a lower gastrointestinal contrast study (which is diagnostic and often therapeutic) is performed in collaboration with our pediatric radiologists to treat inspissated meconium. The fourth quality improvement practice is routine use of probiotics for all infants born less than 33 weeks of gestation (introduced in 2015), driven largely by the Canadian[26] and Australian[27] experience. A probiotic blend is initiated once an infant has a corrected age greater than 23 weeks PMA, a chronological age greater than 3 days, and is tolerating greater than 6 mL/day enteral feedings. The incidence of NEC in inborn, very low birth weight infants at our NICU had ranged between 3% and 6% prior to 2015 and has since ranged from 1% to 3% with no episodes of probiotic-related sepsis. These practices allow us to maintain intestinal health while maximizing the growth and nutrition of the infant.

APPROACH TO SKINCARE

The immature and highly fragile nature of the skin in infants born at 22 weeks' gestation presents 2 key issues: (1) skin breakdown from routine and gentle handling, and (2) difficulties with securing catheters and monitoring leads that are crucial for the care of these infants. See **Box 1** for our approach to skincare. Skin breakdown, even with meticulous care, can increase the risk of infection, including fungal infections. These infants are therefore placed on prophylactic fluconazole for the first 2 weeks of life during the process of epidermal keratinization.

In conclusion, the approach to the care of the 22-week infant at the University of Iowa reflects an interplay of collective awareness of the developmental vulnerability of immature organs, a rigorous approach to monitoring and maintenance of biological homeostasis, recognition of the importance of diagnostic precision and judicious use of therapies, and cohesive team performance.

CLINICS CARE POINTS

- The care of infants born at 22 weeks' gestation begins with the provision of maternal antenatal steroids at 21 5/7 weeks by the MFM physicians.
- The initial care of these infants is more similar than different to that of more mature preterm infants (24–25 weeks' gestation), with special attention to thermal, fluid, cardiovascular and respiratory support.
- Neurodevelopment and neuroprotection should be leading principles of all aspects of the care of infants born at 22 weeks.
- Intubation with a 2.0 endotracheal tube is often needed with these infants and is compatible with adequate CO_2 removal using HVJV.
- These infants use terminal respiratory bronchioles for gas exchange, relatively non-dispensible units that respond to over inflation with pulmonary interstitial emphysema.
- Fluid management depends on environmental/thermal management and must be individually tailored and monitored quite frequently with these infants.
- Evaluating the hemodynamic significance of the PDA, and treating when necessary, decreases mortality and morbidity in these infants
- Probiotics and breastmilk work synergistically (and safely) to prevent intestinal dysbiosis, thus decreasing the risk of NEC.

POTENTIAL CONFLICTS OF INTEREST

The authors declare no conflicts of interest.

FINANCIAL DISCLOSURE

The authors have no relevant financial relationships to disclose.

ACKNOWLEDGMENTS

The authors would like to acknowledge the contributions of Dr Regan Giesinger to this manuscript, a dear colleague who recently lost her battle with cancer. The authors would also like to thank the following for their helpful comments and suggestions after reviewing the manuscript: Brady J. A. Thomas MD, Cassandra

K. Palasiewicz DNP, ARNP, Emily A. Spellman MSN, RNC,[4] and Susan J Carlson, MMSc, RD.

REFERENCES

1. Watkins PL, Dagle JM, Bell EF, et al. Outcomes at 18 to 22 Months of corrected age for infants born at 22 to 25 Weeks of gestation in a center practicing active management. J Pediatr 2020;217:52–8.e1.
2. Brion LPBE, Raghuveer TS. Vitamin E supplementation for prevention of morbidity and mortality in preterm infants. Cochrane Database Syst Rev 2003;4:CD003665.
3. Agren J, Sjörs G, Sedin G. Ambient humidity influences the rate of skin barrier maturation in extremely preterm infants. J Pediatr 2006;148(5):613–7.
4. Segar DE, Segar EK, Harshman LA, et al. Physiological approach to sodium supplementation in preterm infants. Am J Perinatol 2018;35(10):994–1000.
5. Elgin TG, Stanford AH, Klein JM. First intention high-frequency jet ventilation for periviable infants. Curr Opin Pediatr 2022;34(2):165–9.
6. Berger JN, Elgin TG, Dagle JM, et al. Survival and short-term respiratory outcomes of <750 g infants initially intubated with 2.0 mm vs. 2.5 mm endotracheal tubes. J Perinatol 2022;42(2):202–8.
7. Dagle JM, Rysavy MA, Hunter SK, et al. Cardiorespiratory management of infants born at 22 weeks' gestation: the Iowa approach. Semin Perinatol 2022;46(1):151545.
8. Chawla S, Natarajan G, Shankaran S, et al. Markers of successful extubation in extremely preterm infants, and morbidity after failed extubation. J Pediatr 2017;189:113–9.e2.
9. Rios DR, Bhattacharya S, Levy PT, et al. Circulatory insufficiency and hypotension related to the ductus arteriosus in neonates. Front Pediatr 2018;6:F474.
10. Giesinger RE, Rios DR, Chatmethakul T, et al. Impact of early hemodynamic screening on extremely preterm outcomes in a high-performance center. Am J Respir Crit Care Med 2023;208(3):290–300.
11. Hooper LV, Midtvedt T, Gordon JI. How host-microbial interactions shape the nutrient environment of the mammalian intestine. Annu Rev Nutr 2002;22:283–307.
12. Cho I, Blaser MJ. The human microbiome: at the interface of health and disease. Nat Rev Genet 2012;13(4):260–70.
13. Stanford AH, Gong H, Noonan M, et al. A direct comparison of mouse and human intestinal development using epithelial gene expression patterns. Pediatr Res 2019. https://doi.org/10.1038/s41390-019-0472-y.
14. Sanderson IR, Walker A, NetLibrary Inc. Development of the gastrointestinal tract. B C Decker; 1999:xii, 324 p. http://www.netLibrary.com/urlapi.asp?action=summary&v=1&bookid=22435.
15. McElroy SJ, Weitkamp JH. Innate immunity in the small intestine of the preterm infant. NeoReviews 2011;12(9):e517–26.
16. Henning SJ. Ontogeny of enzymes in the small intestine. Annu Rev Physiol 1985;47:231–45.
17. Heida FH, Beyduz G, Bulthuis ML, et al. Paneth cells in the developing gut: when do they arise and when do they immune competent? Pediatr Res 2016. https://doi.org/10.1038/pr.2016.67.
18. Battersby C, Santhalingam T, Costeloe K, et al. Incidence of neonatal necrotising enterocolitis in high-income countries: a systematic review. Arch Dis Child Fetal Neonatal Ed 2018;103(2):F182–9.

19. Patel RM, Kandefer S, Walsh MC, et al. Causes and timing of death in extremely premature infants from 2000 through 2011. N Engl J Med 2015;372(4):331–40.
20. Neu J, Walker WA. Necrotizing enterocolitis. Review. N Engl J Med 2011;364(3): 255–64.
21. Lin PW, Nasr TR, Stoll BJ. Necrotizing enterocolitis: recent scientific advances in pathophysiology and prevention. Semin Perinatol 2008;32(2):70–82.
22. Hackam DJ, Sodhi CP, Good M. New insights into necrotizing enterocolitis: from laboratory observation to personalized prevention and treatment. J Pediatr Surg 2019;54(3):398–404.
23. Nolan LS, Rimer JM, Good M. The role of human milk oligosaccharides and probiotics on the neonatal microbiome and risk of necrotizing enterocolitis: a narrative review. Nutrients 2020;12(10).
24. Nolan LS, Wynn JL, Good M. Exploring clinically-relevant experimental models of neonatal shock and necrotizing enterocolitis. Shock 2020;53(5):596–604.
25. Shah J, Singhal N, da Silva O, et al. Intestinal perforation in very preterm neonates: risk factors and outcomes. J perinatology 2015;35(8):595–600.
26. Janvier A, Malo J, Barrington KJ. Cohort study of probiotics in a North American neonatal intensive care unit. J Pediatr 2014;164(5):980–5.
27. Jacobs SE, Tobin JM, Opie GF, et al. Probiotic effects on late-onset sepsis in very preterm infants: a randomized controlled trial. Pediatrics 2013;132(6):1055–62.

Couplet Care—The Next Frontier of Care in the Newborn Intensive Care Unit

Robert D. White, MD

KEYWORDS

- Couplet care • NICU design • Family-centered care

KEY POINTS

- Separation of babies and mothers shortly after birth is a vestige of obstetric care practices implemented in the 1950s; it was abolished in most newborn nurseries in the 1980s but has persisted in newborn intensive care units (NICUs) for reasons that no longer have scientific or financial merit.
- Several pioneering level II, III, and IV NICUs have demonstrated that couplet care can be provided safely, efficiently, and with a high level of family and caregiver satisfaction.
- Planning for couplet care in the NICU requires the inclusion of families as well as neonatal and obstetric caregivers and should incorporate site visits and extensive simulation activities.

The design and operation of newborn intensive care unit (NICU) care is inextricably tied to the period of time in which NICUs were first introduced. Major advances in respiratory support, incubator design, and nutritional interventions occurred in the early 1970s, making NICU care feasible on a large scale at a time when normal newborn care was being provided in large congregate nurseries where babies were kept for observation while their mothers recovered during the postpartum period in a separate area. The familiar image of fathers peering at their newborn infants through a large viewing window is iconic and representative of the cultural norm at the time of separating babies from their parents in the first days after birth. There were several reasons for this practice, but perhaps most notable was the notion that newborn babies need to be kept in a clean environment, something that was not considered possible in the care of their parents. NICUs were introduced in this period, often starting as small rooms off the main nursery area. As NICU care became increasingly sophisticated and successful, NICU populations grew exponentially, ultimately requiring new spaces that were, like the old spaces, designed and operated with parents largely

Regional Newborn Program, Beacon Children's Hospital, 615 North Michigan Street, South Bend, IN 46601, USA
E-mail address: Robert.White@pediatrix.com

Crit Care Nurs Clin N Am 36 (2024) 35–39
https://doi.org/10.1016/j.cnc.2023.08.002
0899-5885/24/© 2023 Elsevier Inc. All rights reserved.

ccnursing.theclinics.com

excluded. These were also congregated spaces, initially without enough room for parents to comfortably visit at the bedside for longer than a few minutes—which was as long as many NICUs were willing to allow them to stay anyway, given that parents were seen as a potential source of serious infections. The use of breast milk was frowned upon because studies had suggested that it was nutritionally inferior to specialized formulas developed for premature infants, so parents were not even allowed this surrogate opportunity with their infant.

In the 1980s, a trend began and rapidly spread to reunite healthy newborn babies with their parents. Congregate newborn nurseries were largely abandoned, and efforts were made to keep families together throughout the perinatal experience—except in the NICU, where multibed NICU design was still considered desirable, even essential. No studies were ever performed that documented the superiority of open-design NICUs, although to some extent, they were indeed essential until extensive electronic monitoring eliminated the need for at least the pretense of "constant observation." By 1990, though, caregivers had begun to rely on technology to provide continuous feedback on an infant's status, making multibed NICUs much more difficult to justify, although they persist in some hospitals to the present day.

The concept of caring for at least some NICU babies in private "single-family" rooms was introduced in the 1990s[1] but its adoption was slow, with only a few NICUs embracing this concept for the next 20 years. Even these rooms, though, were not intended to provide couplet care while the mother was still a patient; it was not until 2017 that NICUs in Sweden, Indiana, and Connecticut were opened that kept babies and mothers together throughout the NICU experience. The success of this concept has led to another innovative phase in NICU care with increasing numbers of couplet care NICUs being opened each year. Because couplet care has significant design and operational needs, many NICUs have to wait until they can undertake major renovations or build a new facility to implement couplet care.

There are now dozens of couplet care NICUs in the United States, sufficient to demonstrate the safety and financial viability of this care. It has been difficult for some clinicians to support the change to couplet care without large randomized controlled trials (RCTs) demonstrating its superiority to open-bay NICU design but it is important to remember that (1) there were no previous studies that established open-bay design as optimal and (2) doing a proper RCT comparison between open-bay and couplet care NICU settings presents major, probably insurmountable hurdles. Three of the early level IV NICUs with couplet care have recently reported their experience,[2,3] confirming the benefits of this approach for both babies and their parents. In this article, we will review both the design and operational considerations necessary for the successful adoption of couplet care when planning for a new NICU.

DESIGN CONSIDERATIONS FOR COUPLET CARE NEWBORN INTENSIVE CARE UNITS

Couplet care requires design changes for a relatively small portion of a NICU because it is only intended for the care of a mother and baby while the mother is still a patient, so this section will not describe features of the NICU not directly related to couplet care. For example, after the mother is discharged, the baby may then be moved to a single-family room or to a multibed open bay room; adoption of couplet care does not require a commitment to one or the other strategy for further care of the baby after the mother has been discharged and examples of both models as well as a hybrid solution all exist.

Rooms designed to care for a baby who may need a high level of NICU care and the baby's mother should be 30.7 meters squared or larger in order to provide sufficient space around each bedside for high levels of care. Many hospitals that offer couplet care do not admit mothers to the NICU who have significant monitoring needs following delivery, such as continued infusion of magnesium sulfate or respiratory support, but even routine postpartum care requires generous clearances around the mother's bed.[4] The baby's bed should also have sufficient clearance for multiple support items such as respirators and pumps, as well as space to provide advanced care and interventions such as intubation and placement of invasive catheters or chest tubes. Because the mother is an adult patient, the room must have access to daylight and a bathroom; it should also have space for the presence of at least 2 other family members or visitors. Because mothers may need/appreciate privacy at times, these bed positions are usually separated by a curtain; the typical arrangement would be to put the mother's bed closest to the window and bathroom and the baby's bed closest to the entrance door so that caregivers would not need to pass through the mother's space to reach the baby.

Monitoring capability and space for support equipment at the infant's bed position should be appropriate for the highest level of care; this may not be necessary for the mother's bed position if admitting mothers with ongoing medical complications is not planned to occur in the couplet care space. These needs are described in greater detail in the Facilities Guidelines Institute (FGI) Guidelines[4] and the Recommended Standards for Newborn ICU Design.[5]

In some hospitals, NICU couplet care is provided in the Obstetric suite; space requirements for the room are similar, although operational considerations may vary, as described in the next section. A third variant of couplet care provides bed positions for multiple mothers and babies in the same congregate room; again, many of the space and monitoring requirements at each bedside will be similar but logistical considerations will vary. Further variations exist; for example, in some hospitals, couplet care is only offered for babies who require intermediate levels of care, whereas babies who require critical care may not be considered eligible for care in a couplet care room. The key factor for planners to consider is what they want their hospital's capability to be in future years. It is possible, for example, to start providing couplet NICU care for only the most stable NICU babies and then expand the service in future years but this can only be accomplished if sufficient space and rooms are available for such an expansion of care.

OPERATIONAL CONSIDERATIONS FOR COUPLET CARE

There are 2 basic approaches to the care of the mother–baby couplet in a NICU: A single nurse can care for both patients, or each patient can have their own specialty nurse. In either case, the nurse may or may not have an assignment that includes the care of other patients, primarily depending on acuity levels and proximity of the patients.

Obviously, some NICU babies can require 1:1 nursing care; these infants may or may not be considered appropriate for couplet care, although several hospitals providing couplet care in their NICUs have demonstrated that such care can be provided in a couplet setting without compromising the infant's care or causing undue distress or disruption to the mother.

The largest operational challenge usually lies in accommodating the needs of the "non-hosting" team. If the couplet care rooms are located in the NICU, the NICU caregivers will have all their support needs readily at hand but obstetric providers can feel like "outsiders" whose needs may not be so readily anticipated and met. Similarly, if couplet care is provided in the obstetric suite, the babies' caregivers may struggle to feel fully supported. It is crucial that these challenges be addressed well in advance of a move to couplet care. Often, a first step would be to provide a very rudimentary form of couplet care in an existing space; for example, a 34-week infant who would ordinarily be transferred to the NICU could receive care along with its mother in a postpartum area modified for this purpose, or that couplet could receive their care in the NICU, again in a space specially modified for that purpose so that teams could begin to anticipate their needs in a full-scale couplet care facility and begin to build the teamwork and expertise that would be required for successful transition.

CLINICS CARE POINTS: PLANNING AN NEWBORN INTENSIVE CARE UNIT WITH COUPLET CARE FEATURES

- The composition of the planning team is crucial. Obviously, families with NICU experience should be integral partners. Regardless of whether the physical location of these rooms is in the NICU or in the obstetric suite, representatives of both services must be on an equal footing.

- Site visits to hospitals currently offering couplet care are crucial so that lessons learned, both positive and negative, can be considered in the new plan.

- An extensive simulation sequence is essential, progressing ultimately to mock care scenarios in fully equipped physical spaces. Couplet care will require new considerations that may not be obvious until simulations in a comparable space are conducted. For example, does the new design facilitate easy movement between the baby and mother's beds so that, when appropriate, the baby can be skin-to-skin with the mother even when connected to monitors, IV pumps, and respiratory support? How would couplet care be provided to twins?

- As noted previously, one aspect of the simulation process would be, when possible, to introduce a modified form of couplet care in an existing space. This can be valuable to inform planning needs but also to build acceptance and enthusiasm for the concept as caregivers experience reduced anxiety and increased gratification with their experience in the new model of care.

- Visionary planning is essential—the team must try to imagine how care might look different in the 20 years or more of the unit's life span, both in terms of higher technology capabilities, but also in terms of an increasing trend toward nurturing care in which babies may spend far more time in the arms of their parents or a caregiver than they do now. These strong, definite, but very disparate trends must be anticipated as clearly as possible, especially to the extent that one (better technology) will make the other (more nurturing and personal care) increasingly safe and feasible.

- A correlate to the previous point is that nearly all assumptions about how we provide care should be challenged and carefully considered. One needs only to consider how dramatically our care of critically ill newborns has changed over the previous 30 to 40 years to realize the value of anticipating future developments. One way paradigm-shifting changes can be missed is by holding on to assumptions that most care will proceed similarly to what it "always" has. A few examples of changes that could occur in the next 30 to 40 years will help to illustrate the importance of this point:
  - Could oxygen delivery and CO_2 removal for an infant with extremely immature or injured lungs be accomplished by directly oxygenating the blood without using the lungs, such as when the infant is in utero? Research may produce an "artificial placenta" and/or the feasibility of extra-corporeal membrane oxygenator (ECMO) for increasingly tiny babies.
  - Could ventilators, IV pumps, and other technology be managed continuously by computer-based algorithms so that ventilator support, for example, would constantly be adjusted based on moment-to-moment data provided by saturation, CO_2, and blood pressure monitors, thereby changing the clinician's role to periodically adjusting the algorithm rather than adjusting the settings?

○ Could all of these things happen while the infant is in the arms of his/her parent or caregiver rather than in a warmer or an incubator?

○ Ultrasound and MRI are currently used primarily to provide structural information, but they may become much more valuable for providing ongoing physiologic data, meaning their space and access requirements will need to be anticipated.

○ Although these examples may seem far-fetched, considering that care may trend in those directions may help avoid building a NICU that is obsolete far before it is structurally unfit. It will be apparent, too, that these changes will affect not only structural decisions but also the role of the nurse, respiratory therapist, and other bedside providers.

SUMMARY

Couplet care may affect only a small portion of the NICU space and personnel but, its adoption is likely to drive a much deeper consideration of the needs of the family unit and how we interact with our obstetric colleagues, aspects of neonatal care that are likely to change dramatically during the decades-long life span of a given NICU.

DISCLOSURE

The author has no commercial or financial conflicts of interest and did not receive any funding for this article.

REFERENCES

1. White RD, Whitman TL. Design of ICU's (letter to editor). Pediatrics 1992;89:1267.
2. Klemming S, Lillieskold S, Arwehed S, et al. Mother-Newborn couplet care: Nordic experiences of organization, models and practice. J Perinatol 2023;43(Suppl).
3. Redmond B, Gambardella T, Bruno CJ. Reimagination through renovation: Incorporating couplet care in a level IV academic NICU. J Perinatol 2023;43(Suppl).
4. Facilities Guidelines Institute. Guidelines for Design and Construction of Hospitals, 2022 Edition. The Facility Guidelines Institute.
5. White RD. Consensus Committee on, Recommended design Standards for advanced neonatal care. Recommended standards for newborn ICU design, 10th edition, J Perinatol 2023;43:Suppl, (in press).

Understanding Near-Infrared Spectroscopy
An Update

Terri Marin, PhD, NNP-BC, FAAN, FANNP, FNAP[a],*, James Moore, MD, PhD[b]

KEYWORDS

- Near-infrared spectroscopy • NIRS • Perfusion • Prematurity

KEY POINTS

- Near-infrared spectroscopy (NIRS) is a novel technology that uses infrared light to noninvasively and continuously measure regional oxygen extraction in real time at the bedside.
- NIRS serves as a surrogate marker for end-organ perfusion, making it a valuable adjunct to routine cardiovascular monitoring in neonatal research.
- The device can detect minute changes in cerebral, intestinal, and kidney tissue beds, making it a useful tool in monitoring multiple conditions affecting premature infants frequently associated with hypoperfusion.
- Early detection of tissue-specific perfusion alterations through NIRS may significantly improve the clinician's ability to intervene and prevent further deterioration in premature infants.
- NIRS has potential applications in neonatal care, enabling timely interventions and improving outcomes by closely monitoring regional oxygen extraction and tissue perfusion.

INTRODUCTION

Near-infrared spectroscopy (NIRS) was introduced in 1977 and is a noninvasive technology capable of continuously measuring regional tissue oxygenation at the bedside.[1] When used as an adjunct to routine cardiovascular monitoring, NIRS provides complementary insight into tissue-specific oxygenation changes, serving as a surrogate marker for end-organ perfusion.[2] Research in neonatology has demonstrated that simultaneous NIRS evaluation of cerebral, mesenteric, and kidney oxygenation contributes to early recognition of potential and actual tissue ischemia that may not be readily reflected in current routine bedside monitoring modalities, such as urine output, lactate

[a] Department of Nursing Science, Augusta University, College of Nursing, 1120 15th Street, EC-4350, Augusta, GA 30912, USA; [b] Department of Pediatrics, Division of Neonatology, University of Connecticut School of Medicine, 10 Columbus Boulevard, Hartford, CT 06106, USA
* Corresponding author.
E-mail address: tmarin@augusta.edu

Crit Care Nurs Clin N Am 36 (2024) 41–50
https://doi.org/10.1016/j.cnc.2023.08.001
0899-5885/24/© 2023 Elsevier Inc. All rights reserved.
ccnursing.theclinics.com

levels, pulse oximetry, and blood pressure.[3–5] Because multiple conditions that affect premature infants are frequently associated with hypoperfusion, methods to detect early alterations in perfusion that are tissue-targeted may substantially improve the clinician's ability to intervene and prevent further deterioration. The purpose of this article is to provide a comprehensive overview of NIRS principles, its use in neonatology, and how current research demonstrates the benefit of this novel technology.

Near-Infrared Spectroscopy Principles

NIRS technology uses infrared light wavelengths to measure the difference between oxyhemoglobin and deoxyhemoglobin, reflecting oxygen uptake in the respective tissue beds being monitored. Depending on the NIRS platform used, infrared light is emitted at approximately 1 to 3 cm depth and is absorbed by chromophores, such as hemoglobin and cytochrome aa3. The amount of light absorbed depends on chromophore concentration and oxygenated state.[6,7] The most widely used device in neonatology, the INVOS 7100 system (Medtronic Inc., Boulder, CO),[2,7] emits 2 infrared light wavelengths of different depths from the sensor, one shallow (730 nm) and one deep (810 nm), that is received by 2 optodes on the opposite end of the sensor (**Fig. 1**).[6] The displayed value on the monitor screen subtracts the shallow reading (peripheral) from the deep reading producing a tissue-specific measure of oxygen uptake, known as the regional oxygen saturation (rSO_2). In comparison to pulse oximetry, which requires pulsatile blood flow to measure the oxyhemoglobin content in arterial blood, NIRS measures the difference between oxygenated and deoxygenated hemoglobin in the tissue of interest, where oxygen contribution is approximately 75% venous, 20% arterial, and 5% capillary.[8] Therefore, the rSO_2 value reflects the amount of oxygen absorbed within the tissue bed relative to the amount delivered (**Fig. 2**), reflecting a venous-weighted saturation level. NIRS systems are capable of simultaneous real-time multiple organ (regional) monitoring which is unique to the neonate. Concurrent cerebral, kidney, and mesenteric monitoring allows the evaluation of differential, tissue-specific oxygen delivery and uptake during periods of hemodynamic instability.[9]

Measures of perfusion

Hypotension leading to systemic hypoperfusion is commonly associated with many conditions of prematurity, such as sepsis, patent ductus arteriosus, intraventricular hemorrhage, and necrotizing enterocolitis (NEC).[10–12] Similarly, critically ill term infants with congenital cardiac disease, hypoxic-ischemic encephalopathy, or those requiring extracorporeal membrane oxygenation (ECMO) are at risk for hemodynamic instability.[13,14] Conventional markers of perfusion routinely assessed in critically ill neonates are capillary refill, color changes, strength of peripheral pulse, urinary output, and blood pressure. Laboratory measures to evaluate perfusion alterations include

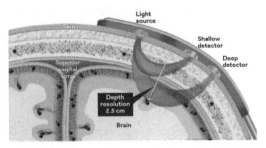

Fig. 1. NIRS wavelength depth measured by cerebral sensor. (©2024 Medtronic. All rights reserved. Used with the permission of Medtronic.)

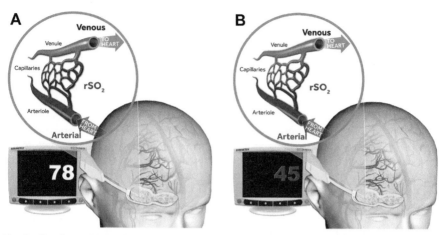

Fig. 2. *(A, B)* INVOS 5100C measuring rSO$_2$ in cerebral tissue-bed. *(A)* Adequately oxygenated blood from the heart (SaO$_2$) enters the arteriole to capillary bed where oxygen extraction occurs. The arteriole with the red SaO$_2$ extends through two-thirds of the capillary bed going from red to purple to blue (this is to illustrate adequate O$_2$ delivery) with the vein remaining blue. The INVOS monitor screen shows an rSO$_2$ reading of 78% as an example. Diagram *B* shows a thinner arteriole with red SaO$_2$; however, it turns purple to blue almost immediately as it enters the capillaries from the thinner arteriole and shows an rSO$_2$ of 45, to illustrate that the tissue has extracted much more O$_2$ because blood flow is reduced and oxygen extraction is greater. (©2024 Medtronic. All rights reserved. Used with the permission of Medtronic.)

blood pH, lactate levels, and kidney function biomarkers such as creatinine. However, the temporal relationship for when these measures may indicate organ-specific perfusion is highly variable (**Fig. 3**) and may significantly delay prompt recognition and treatment. During periods of hemodynamic stability, oxygen delivery and extraction are relatively constant to meet tissue metabolic demands. However, when homeostasis is compromised and oxygen delivery is reduced, oxygen extraction begins to increase

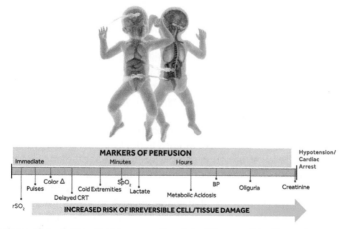

Fig. 3. Markers of perfusion that increase the risk of irreversible tissue damage over time. (©2024 Medtronic. All rights reserved. Used with the permission of Medtronic.)

to meet tissue oxygen requirements. With prolonged or sustained oxygen depletion, a critical oxygenation point is reached where maximum oxygen extraction occurs, and tissue needs are insufficiently met by delivery.[8] For NIRS tracings, this translates as sharp declines in rSO_2 readings, indicating the tissue being monitored is experiencing oxygen deprivation.

Numerous studies have shown that rSO_2 measurement changes occur in real time, when actual tissue oxygenation is affected, and are often the first measure of perfusion status to indicate tissue-specific hypoxia.[4,15–19] This earlier warning can prompt further clinical investigation into the underlying cause(s), which can halt ischemia progression and prevent tissue damage and death. For example, a septic premature infant being monitored with cerebral and kidney NIRS who develops ischemic acute kidney injury (AKI) may exhibit acute and/or prolonged drops in rSO_2 values before changes in cerebral rSO_2 due to preferential shunting to the brain during hypoperfusion. Elevated serum creatinine and oliguria are late findings in AKI and may not be apparent for 24 to 48 hours following the initial ischemic insult.[20] A routine perfusion assessment may not readily identify kidney-specific perfusion changes until lactate build-up and metabolic acidosis occur (see **Fig. 3**). In this scenario, the clinician is alerted to kidney-specific perfusion changes at the time they occur and can adjust the neonate's treatment plan accordingly and potentially avert AKI development.

Normative regional oxygen saturation data

To accurately interpret rSO_2 data, expected reference ranges for each organ region monitored must be known. Data have shown that baseline rSO_2 values will vary dependent on gestation and postnatal age, as well as the NIRS platform used.[21–23] Because of these differences, NIRS is intended for continuous trend monitoring over time.[23] Organ oxygen utilization is determined by metabolic demand and hemodynamic stability. The variability of rSO_2 in cerebral beds is approximately 3%, although slightly higher variability is seen in the kidney (6%) and is highest in mesenteric beds (16%).[24] Cerebral tissue has consistent metabolic demands, whereas the demand for oxygen in kidney and mesenteric tissues fluctuates depending on metabolic activity. In kidney beds, data suggest that rSO_2 values are higher immediately after birth and gradually decline and plateau around the end of the first week of life.[21] Mesenteric values typically begin midrange with a modest decline until approximately 7 to 10 days, followed by a gradual increase back to midrange.[22,25]

It is important to understand that NIRS only measures oxygen uptake in vascularized regions; nonvascular structures/spaces do not contribute to rSO_2 readings and may explain the regional variability and normative value differences.[24] The brain has a relatively higher and more constant metabolic requirement than somatic organs; therefore, cerebral rSO_2 values are typically lower than somatic readings during homeostasis, reflecting greater oxygen uptake (or extraction) in tissue beds. Lower variability in cerebral beds suggests blood flow autoregulation with steady levels of oxygen consumption.[24] A multicenter observational study determined that mean cerebral rSO_2 was 65% ($\pm$1%) in extremely low birthweight (ELBW) infants (n = 124) during the first week of life.[26] Other earlier studies suggest cerebral rSO_2 range of greater than 60% to 70% to be ideal, although sample sizes in these studies were small.[22,27,28]

The rSO_2 trends seen in kidney beds during the first week of life may be related to blood flow and oxygenation changes that occur during the transition from intrauterine to extrauterine life.[21] In premature infants, roughly 3% to 4% of total cardiac output reaches the kidney, which gradually increases to 10% by the end of the first week reflecting reduced kidney resistance and stabilizing function.[22,29] A recent study found that mean kidney rSO_2 ranges begin between 75% and 80% and gradually decline and plateau to 55% to 65% by day of life 7 for infants less than 32 weeks' gestation; importantly, infants of lower gestational age have lower overall kidney rSO$_2$ baselines.[21]

Multiple factors most likely explain the high rSO$_2$ variation in mesenteric beds, as this region contains fluid, stool, gas, and fluctuant tissue (peristalsis). In addition, intestinal oxygenation demand depends on digestion intervals associated with bolus feedings.[30] A large multicenter study found mesenteric rSO$_2$ means in ELBW infants (n = 124) during the first week of life shows higher initial rSO$_2$ levels with gradual stabilization to 45.4 $\pm$ 21% by day of life (DOL) 7.[26] For infants less than 32 weeks' gestation (n = 220), similar patterns were found with mesenteric rSO$_2$ beginning at 48.2 $\pm$ 16%, declining to 37% $\pm$ 17% on DOL 5 plateauing to 44% $\pm$ 16% on DOL 7.[31]

Correlative studies

To validate the clinical usefulness and validity of NIRS, many studies have examined the correlation between cerebral rSO$_2$ (CrSO$_2$) and somatic rSO$_2$ values to other noninvasive and invasive monitoring measures. Aortic blood flow measured by echocardiogram in infants less than 29 weeks' gestation has been correlated with CrSO$_2$ (preductal flow) and kidney saturations (KrSO$_2$) (postductal flow) when observing aortic flow from the substernal view but not subcostal view.[32] Data also show strong correlation between SvO$_2$ and CrSO$_2$ in children undergoing single-ventricle palliative surgery ($r^2 = 0.45$; $P < .0001$).[33] Another study found a strong correlation between CrSO$_2$ and SvO$_2$ ($r^2 = 0.58$; $P = .008$), and marginally significant correlation between KrSO$_2$ and SvO$_2$ ($r^2 = 0.38$; $P = .09$) in children undergoing corrective cardiac surgery.[34] In a piglet study simulating veno-arterial ECMO, CrSO$_2$ correlated well with SvO$_2$ ($r^2 = 0.59$; $P = .001$), and during induced hypoxia, this correlation became stronger ($r^2 = 0.75$; $P < .001$), suggesting that trend CrSO$_2$ monitoring during ECMO provides a reasonably accurate reflection of hemodynamic neurologic changes.[35] In a large cohort study of critically ill infants (n = 155), CrSO$_2$ significantly correlated to arterial oxygen saturation (SaO$_2$) ($r = 0.254$, $P < .001$) and SvO$_2$ ($r = 0.32$, $P < .001$).[36] Kidney oxygenation has shown strong correlation to SaO$_2$ ($r = 0.32$; $P < .01$) and capillary oxygen saturation ($r = 0.26$; $P = .03$) but not SvO$_2$ ($r = 0.07$; $P = .74$).[37] Data from these studies clearly support that tissue oxygenation measured by NIRS provides a reliable trend assessment that reflects end-organ perfusion.

Clinical use in neonatology

During the past decade, more than 150 studies have incorporated NIRS technology to assess alteration in regional oxygenation associated with various conditions of prematurity, commonly used therapeutics, and routine care. Cerebral oxygenation (CrSO$_2$) has been the most widely studied aspect; however, studies examining kidney and mesenteric oxygenation are gaining substantial attention.

Historically, cerebral NIRS monitoring has primarily been used in infants undergoing cardiothoracic surgery to assess for neurologic insult secondary to cerebral hypoxia.[18,38,39] Because critically ill infants, especially those born prematurely, are at significant risk for neurodevelopmental delay, recent cerebral oxygenation studies have expanded their focus. Determining a CrSO$_2$ threshold for clinical assessment may be the most useful implication. Studies have reported that a CrSO$_2$ cutoff value of 50% to 55% may correctly identify preterm infants at greatest risk for adverse neurologic outcomes.[40,41] Alderstein and colleagues evaluated CrSO$_2$ during the first 72 hours of life in infants less than 32 weeks' gestation (n = 734) and found those with readings less than 55% were associated with increased numbers of severe IVH (Grade III/IV) and adverse cognitive outcomes at 24 months of age.[40] Similarly, Chock and colleagues evaluated

CrSO$_2$ during the first 96 hours of life in infants less than 1260 g (n = 103) and found that a threshold of 50% readily identifies those at risk for adverse outcomes (mortality, severe IVH, or PVL) with a sensitivity of 52%, specificity of 87%, and negative predictive value of 88%.[41]

Multisite simultaneous NIRS monitoring can be a valuable approach to evaluating differential regional oxygen distribution and uptake in critically ill infants.[42] Hoffman and colleagues examined cerebral and kidney NIRS data and routine cardiovascular measures from 194 infants following stage 1 palliation for hypoplastic left heart syndrome to determine which combination of measures most reliably predicted survivability.[19] Multivariate logistic regression modeling revealed that heart rate, mean arterial pressure, and both cerebral and kidney rSO$_2$ were the best predictors of survivability at 48 hours postoperatively (area under the curve = 0.834; $P <$ .0001).[19] Infants with hemodynamically significant patent ductus arteriosus (hsPDA) are at risk for reduced systemic perfusion to the brain, kidneys, and gut due to bidirectional blood shunting at the pulmonary artery level.[43–45] Thus, differential and continual regional rSO$_2$ monitoring with NIRS provides distributive oxygenation variation and can alert the bedside clinician to potential ischemic events that may not be readily apparent in conventional cardiovascular monitoring.

Using NIRS to evaluate for perfusion-related kidney injury among premature infants has gained momentum during the past decade.[2] Several conditions of prematurity are associated with kidney hypoxia that may lead to AKI, such as hsPDA, bronchopulmonary dysplasia, NEC, sepsis, anemia, and the use of nephrotoxic medications.[2] Multiple studies have evaluated if these conditions are associated with diminished KrSO$_2$, and the results are mixed. For example, data from one study suggest KrSO$_2$ less than 66% were associated with hsPDA,[45] whereas others found no difference in KrSO$_2$ between infants with and without hsPDA.[44,46,47] Cyclooxygenase inhibitors are commonly used to pharmacologically manage hsPDA; however, these agents (ibuprofen and indomethacin) produce ductal closure through prostaglandin reduction and subsequent constriction, which may also induce kidney hypoperfusion, especially if dysfunction already exists.[48] In one small study (n = 38) analyzing regional oxygenation in infants less than 32 weeks' gestation receiving either ibuprofen (n = 20) or indomethacin (n = 18), kidney oxygenation was reduced in 36.8% of infants ($P <$ .04) with no significant difference between those who received ibuprofen versus, indomethacin. They further found that higher beginning KrSO$_2$ baselines were associated with larger reductions 1-hour posttreatment ($P <$ .0001).[48] In contrast, 2 other studies have shown that ibuprofen administration had no effect on kidney oxygenation and was actually associated with improved KrSO$_2$ up to 48 hours following treatment.[46,49,50] These studies concluded that ductal closure eliminated the "ductal steal" phenomenon, triggering increased regional blood flow and oxygen delivery to kidney tissues.

To fully evaluate the influence of kidney hypoxia, AKI incidence must be determined; however, studies including the outcome of AKI are limited. One large study (n = 128) found that infants less than 32 weeks' gestation who developed AKI had significantly lower KrSO$_2$ means on the first day of life compared with those who did not (69.7 ± 11.3 vs 80.4 ± 9.5; $P <$ .001).[5] Another study (n = 100) found that infants who developed AKI had significantly lower KrSO$_2$ on days of life 1 through 4, than those who did not develop AKI.[51] Another smaller study (n = 35) found that infants less than 32 weeks' gestation who developed AKI had significantly lower median KrSO$_2$ than those who did not (32.4% vs 60%; $P <$ .001) during the first week of life and data further suggested that decreases in KrSO$_2$ occurred during the 48-hour period before serum creatinine changes in those with AKI.[52]

Several studies have examined alterations in mesenteric perfusion (mes-rSO$_2$) related to enteral feeding intolerance and packed red blood cell (RBC) transfusions with the intent to identify patterns that indicate an increased risk for NEC. In a small study (n = 17), mes-rSO$_2$ was not influenced by enteral feeding during an RBC transfusion; however, these infants did show negative mes-rSO$_2$ patterns up to 15 hours post-transfusion compared with infants that were not fed during transfusion ($P < .01$).[3] Other studies have shown that infants who develop NEC exhibit persistently decreased mes-rSO$_2$ accompanied by periods of signal dropout, possibly indicating impaired signal detection due to ischemic bowel or accumulation of free air.[4,15,25,53]

SUMMARY

Multiple strategies to incorporate NIRS trend analysis into routine bedside clinical use exist in Neonatology. This novel technology provides a continuous and noninvasive surrogate marker for end-organ perfusion in real time and further allows regional assessment of differential oxygen utilization. Although numerous studies have established NIRS ability to detect low perfusion states associated with multiple conditions of prematurity, further large cohort studies are needed to validate predictive rSO$_2$ thresholds relative to gestational and postnatal age. Existing data confirm that NIRS is capable of enhancing conventional cardiovascular monitoring because it identifies tissue-specific hypoxic events, creating the opportunity for therapeutic intervention to reduce or prevent end-organ damage.

DISCLOSURE

This article will not be submitted to any other journal for consideration. No funding was received for the production of this article. Dr T. Marin provides clinical education on the use of the INVOS device for Medtronic, Inc. Dr J. Moore has no conflicts of interest to disclose. Dr T. Marin composed the initial draft of this article and received subsequent input from Dr J. Moore. Both authors have viewed and approved the final submission of this article version.

REFERENCES

1. Jöbsis FF. Noninvasive, infrared monitoring of cerebral and myocardial oxygen sufficiency and circulatory parameters. Science 1977;198(4323):1264–7.
2. Marin T, Williams BL. Renal oxygenation measured by near-infrared spectroscopy in neonates. Adv Neonatal Care 2020;21(4):256–66.
3. Marin T, Josephson CD, Kosmetatos N, et al. Feeding preterm infants during red blood cell transfusion is associated with a decline in postprandial mesenteric oxygenation. J Pediatr 2014;165(3):464–71.e461.
4. Marin T, Moore JE. Mesenteric oxygenation changes associated with necrotizing enterocolitis and pneumoperitoneum after multiple blood transfusions: a case report. Adv Neonatal Care 2018;18(2):121–7.
5. Bonsante F, Ramful D, Binquet C, et al. Low renal oxygen saturation at near-infrared spectroscopy on the first day of life is associated with developing acute kidney injury in very preterm infants. Neonatology 2019;115(3):198–204.
6. Dullenkopf A, Frey B, Baenziger O, et al. Measurement of cerebral oxygenation state in anaesthetized children using the INVOS 5100 cerebral oximeter. Pediatric Anesthesia 2003;13(5):384–91.
7. Sood BG, McLaughlin K, Cortez J. Near-infrared spectroscopy: applications in neonates. Semin Fetal Neonatal Med 2015;20(3):164–72.

8. Mintzer JP, Moore JE. Regional tissue oxygenation monitoring in the neonatal intensive care unit: evidence for clinical strategies and future directions. Pediatr Res 2019;86(3):296–304.

9. Marin T, Moore J. Understanding near-infrared spectroscopy. Adv Neonatal Care 2011;11(6):382–8.

10. Kharrat A, Jain A. Hemodynamic dysfunction in neonatal sepsis. Pediatr Res 2022;91(2):413–24.

11. Johnson PJ. Hydrocortisone for treatment of hypotension in the newborn. Neonatal Netw 2015;34(1):46–51.

12. Hsu K-H, Nguyen J, Dekom S, et al. Effects of patent ductus arteriosus on organ blood flow in infants born very preterm: a prospective study with serial echocardiography. J Pediatr 2020;216:95–100.e102.

13. Giesinger RE, McNamara PJ. Hemodynamic instability in the critically ill neonate: an approach to cardiovascular support based on disease pathophysiology. Semin Perinatol 2016;40(3):174–88.

14. Zwiers AJ, de Wildt SN, Hop WC, et al. Acute kidney injury is a frequent complication in critically ill neonates receiving extracorporeal membrane oxygenation: a 14-year cohort study. Crit Care 2013;17(4):R151.

15. Marin T, Moore J, Kosmetatos N, et al. Red blood cell transfusion–related necrotizing enterocolitis in very-low-birthweight infants: a near-infrared spectroscopy investigation. Transfusion 2013;53(11):2650–8.

16. Alderliesten T, Lemmers PM, Smarius JJ, et al. Cerebral oxygenation, extraction, and autoregulation in very preterm infants who develop peri-intraventricular hemorrhage. J Pediatr 2013;162(4):698–704.e692.

17. Verhagen EA, Hummel LA, Bos AF, et al. Near-infrared spectroscopy to detect absence of cerebrovascular autoregulation in preterm infants. Clin Neurophysiol 2014;125(1):47–52.

18. Koch HW, Hansen TG. Perioperative use of cerebral and renal near-infrared spectroscopy in neonates: a 24-h observational study. Pediatric Anesthesia 2016;26(2):190–8.

19. Hoffman GM, Ghanayem NS, Scott JP, et al. Postoperative cerebral and somatic near-infrared spectroscopy saturations and outcome in hypoplastic left heart syndrome. Ann Thorac Surg 2017;103(1527–35).

20. Selewski DT, Charlton JR, Jetton JG, et al. Neonatal acute kidney injury. Pediatrics 2015;136(2):e463–73.

21. Marin T, Williams BL, Mansuri A, et al. Renal oxygenation (rSO2) population parameter estimates in premature infants routinely monitored with near-infrared spectroscopy. Adv Neonatal Care 2022;22(4):370–7.

22. McNeill S, Gatenby JC, McElroy S, et al. Normal cerebral, renal and abdominal regional oxygen saturations using near-infrared spectroscopy in preterm infants. J Perinatol 2011;31(1):51–7.

23. Schneider A, Minnich B, Hofstätter E, et al. Comparison of four near-infrared spectroscopy devices shows that they are only suitable for monitoring cerebral oxygenation trends in preterm infants. Acta Paediatr 2014;103(9):934–8.

24. Mintzer JP, Parvez B, Chelala M, et al. Quiescent variability of cerebral, renal, and splanchnic regional tissue oxygenation in very low birth weight neonates. J Neonatal Perinat Med 2014;7(3):199–206.

25. Cortez J, Gupta M, Amaram A, et al. Noninvasive evaluation of splanchnic tissue oxygenation using near-infrared spectroscopy in preterm neonates. J Matern Fetal Neonatal Med 2011;24(4):574–82.

26. Chock VY, Smith E, Tan S, et al. Early brain and abdominal oxygenation in extremely low birth weight infants. Pediatr Res 2022;92(4):1034–41.

27. Petrova A, Mehta R. Near-infrared spectroscopy in the detection of regional tissue oxygenation during hypoxic events in preterm infants undergoing critical care. Pediatr Crit Care Med 2006;7(5):449–54.

28. Lemmers PM, Toet M, van Schelven LJ, et al. Cerebral oxygenation and cerebral oxygen extraction in the preterm infant: the impact of respiratory distress syndrome. Exp Brain Res 2006;173(3):458–67.

29. Nada A, Bonachea EM, Askenazi DJ. Acute kidney injury in the fetus and neonate. Semin Fetal Neonatal Med 2017;22(2):90–7.

30. Martini S, Corvaglia L. Splanchnic NIRS monitoring in neonatal care: rationale, current applications and future perspectives. J Perinatol 2018;38(5):431–43.

31. van der Heide M, Dotinga Baukje M, Stewart RE, et al. Regional splanchnic oxygen saturation for preterm infants in the first week after birth: reference values. Pediatr Res 2021;90(4):882–7.

32. Altit G, Bhombal S, Chock VY. End-organ saturations correlate with aortic blood flow estimates by echocardiography in the extremely premature newborn - an observational cohort study. BMC Pediatr 2021;21(1):312.

33. Tortoriello TA, Stayer SA, Mott AR, et al. A noninvasive estimation of mixed venous oxygen saturation using near-infrared spectroscopy by cerebral oximetry in pediatric cardiac surgery patients. Pediatric Anesthesia 2005;15(6):495–503.

34. Marimón GA, Dockery WK, Sheridan MJ, et al. Near-infrared spectroscopy cerebral and somatic (renal) oxygen saturation correlation to continuous venous oxygen saturation via intravenous oximetry catheter. J Crit Care 2012;27(3):314.e313–8.

35. Tyree K, Tyree M, DiGeronimo R. Correlation of brain tissue oxygen tension with cerebral near-infrared spectroscopy and mixed venous oxygen saturation during extracorporeal membrane oxygenation. Perfusion 2009;24(5):325–31.

36. Weiss M, Dullenkopf A, Kolarova A, et al. Near-infrared spectroscopic cerebral oxygenation reading in neonates and infants is associated with central venous oxygen saturation. Pediatric Anesthesia 2005;15(2):102–9.

37. Harer MW, Gadek L, Rothwell AC, et al. Correlation of Renal Tissue Oxygenation to Venous, Arterial, and Capillary Blood Gas Oxygen Saturation in Preterm Neonates. Am J Perinatol 2023. https://doi.org/10.1055/s-0043-1761296.

38. Hofer A, Haizinger B, Geiselseder G, et al. Monitoring of selective antegrade cerebral perfusion using near infrared spectroscopy in neonatal aortic arch surgery. Eur J Anaesthesiol 2005;22(4):293–8.

39. Gil-Anton J, Redondo S, Garcia Urabayen D, et al. Pilar J. Combined cerebral and renal near-infrared spectroscopy after congenital heart surgery. Pediatr Cardiol 2015;36(6):1173–8.

40. Alderliesten T, van Bel F, van der Aa NE, et al. Low cerebral oxygenation in preterm infants is associated with adverse neurodevelopmental outcome. J Pediatr 2019;207:109–16.e102.

41. Chock VY, Kwon SH, Ambalavanan N, et al. Cerebral oxygenation and autoregulation in preterm infants (early NIRS study). J Pediatr 2020;227:94–100.e101.

42. Hoffman SB, Magder LS, Viscardi RM. Renal versus cerebral saturation trajectories: the perinatal transition in preterm neonates. Pediatr Res 2022;92(5):1437–42.

43. Cohen E, Dix L, Baerts W, et al. Reduction in cerebral oxygenation due to patent ductus arteriosus is pronounced in small-for-gestational-age neonates. Neonatology 2017;111(2):126–32.

44. Petrova A, Bhatt M, Mehta R. Regional tissue oxygenation in preterm born infants in association with echocardiographically significant patent ductus arteriosus. J Perinatol 2011;31(7):460–4.
45. Chock VY, Rose LA, Mante JV, et al. Near-infrared spectroscopy for detection of a significant patent ductus arteriosus. Pediatr Res 2016;80(5):675–80.
46. Guzoglu N, Sari FN, Ozdemir R, et al. Renal and mesenteric tissue oxygenation in preterm infants treated with oral ibuprofen. J Matern Fetal Neonatal Med: The Official Journal Of The European Association Of Perinatal Medicine, The Federation Of Asia And Oceania Perinatal Societies, The International Society Of Perinatal Obstetricians 2014;27(2):197–203.
47. van der Laan ME, Roofthooft MTR, Fries MWA, et al. A hemodynamically significant patent ductus arteriosus does not affect cerebral or renal tissue oxygenation in preterm infants. Neonatology 2016;110(2):141–7.
48. Bhatt M, Petrova A, Mehta R. Does treatment of patent ductus arteriosus with cyclooxygenase inhibitors affect neonatal regional tissue oxygenation? Pediatr Cardiol 2012;33(8):1307–14.
49. Navikienė J, Liubšys A, Viršilas E, et al. Impact of medical treatment of hemodynamically significant patent ductus arteriosus on cerebral and renal tissue oxygenation measured by near-infrared spectroscopy in very low-birth-weight infants. Medicina (Kaunas) 2022;58(4).
50. Arman D, Sancak S, Gursoy T, et al. The association between NIRS and Doppler ultrasonography in preterm infants with patent ductus arteriosus. J Matern Fetal Neonatal Med 2020;33(7):1245–52.
51. Dorum BA, Ozkan H, Cetinkaya M, et al. Regional oxygen saturation and acute kidney injury in premature infants. Pediatr Int 2021;63(3):290–4.
52. Harer MW, Adegboro CO, Richard LJ, et al. Non-invasive continuous renal tissue oxygenation monitoring to identify preterm neonates at risk for acute kidney injury. Pediatr Nephrol 2021;36(6):1617–25.
53. Zabaneh RN, Cleary JP, Lieber CA. Mesentric oxygen saturations in premature twins with and without necrotizing enterocolitis. Ped Crit Care Med 2011;12(6):404–6.

Noninvasive Ventilation

Rangasamy Ramanathan, MBBS, DCH, MD[a],*,
Manoj Biniwale, MBBS, MD[a]

KEYWORDS

- Noninvasive ventilation • Nasal continuous positive airway pressure
- Nasal intermittent positive pressure ventilation • Sigh positive airway pressure
- Bilevel positive airway pressure • Nasal high-frequency oscillatory ventilation
- Nasal high-frequency jet ventilation • Noninvasive neurally adjusted ventilatory assist

KEY POINTS

- Invasive mechanical ventilation is one of the key factors contributing to bronchopulmonary dysplasia.
- Noninvasive ventilation has been shown to decrease the risk of bronchopulmonary dysplasia and mortality compared to invasive mechanical ventilation.
- Among the different modes of noninvasive ventilation, nasal intermittent positive pressure ventilation is superior to nasal continuous positive airway pressure or biphasic modes in decreasing the need for intubation, bronchopulmonary dysplasia, and/or mortality.

SCOPE OF THE PROBLEM

Extremely preterm and low–birth weight (BW) infants often require positive pressure ventilatory support right after they are born or on admission to the neonatal intensive care unit (NICU). Most of these infants have respiratory distress syndrome (RDS) and may need significant respiratory support right from the delivery room. Major long-term morbidities in these infants include bronchopulmonary dysplasia (BPD), need for home oxygen, and abnormal neurodevelopmental outcomes. Several of these infants may have abnormal lung function beyond infancy and a predisposition for respiratory infections requiring hospital admissions in the first years of life. Development of BPD in this population has been linked with long-term adverse pulmonary and neurologic outcomes.[1] Major factors contributing to the long-term injury of the lungs include prolonged invasive mechanical ventilation (IMV) and supplemental oxygen. Even brief periods of IMV result in the release of systemic proinflammatory cytokines, such as interleukin (IL)-8 and tumor necrosis factor alfa, and down-regulation of anti-inflammatory cytokines such as IL-10.[2] Further, systemic inflammation results in a

[a] Division of Neonatology, Department of Pediatrics, Keck School of Medicine of USC, Los Angeles General Medical Center, 1200 North State Street, IRD-820, Los Angeles, CA 90033, USA
* Corresponding author.
E-mail address: ramanath@usc.edu

Crit Care Nurs Clin N Am 36 (2024) 51–67
https://doi.org/10.1016/j.cnc.2023.11.001
0899-5885/24/© 2023 Elsevier Inc. All rights reserved.
ccnursing.theclinics.com

prolonged need for IMV in extremely low–gestational age (GA) infants.[3] Persistent inflammatory state leads to injury to the immature developing lung in preterm infants and subsequent development of BPD. Noninvasive ventilation (NIV) introduced right from the delivery room may significantly impact the outcomes in these vulnerable infants.

RESPIRATORY SUPPORT IN THE DELIVERY ROOM

Many preterm infants need positive pressure ventilation (PPV) support in the delivery room during the fetal-to-neonatal transition when there is an isovolumic transformation of a fluid-filled lung to an air-breathing lung. In preterm infants, a very compliant chest wall and a poorly compliant lung due to surfactant deficiency makes this transition difficult, often needing PPV support. Typically, continuous positive airway pressure (CPAP) is applied using a face mask. In a recent systematic review and meta-analysis of 5 randomized controlled trials (RCTs) including 1225 newborns, investigators concluded that there is little high-quality evidence for choosing a particular type of face mask and suggested that binasal cannula appear to offer some advantages over face masks but need further studies.[4] Schmölzer and colleagues studied resuscitation with a face mask in 56 preterm infants using a respiratory function monitor and found airway obstruction (defined as a 75% decrease in exhaled tidal volume) in 26% of the patients and mask leaks in 51% of the patients.[5] Airway obstruction and mask leaks are very common, especially in very preterm infants making resuscitation and stabilization often unsuccessful. Another study evaluated the effect of face mask application during resuscitation on breathing patterns in 429 preterm infants $\leq$ 32 weeks of GA.

These investigators showed that applying a face mask triggered trigeminocardiac reflex (TCR) leading to apnea in 54% of the infants with associated bradycardia and desaturations. They also concluded that avoiding sensitive areas around the mouth by using alternative interfaces such as nasal prongs might decrease the risk of inducing TCR.[6] Capasso and colleagues performed an RCT comparing nasal cannula (NC) versus face mask for primary neonatal resuscitation in 617 newborn infants and showed that NC as an interface during resuscitation resulted in less need for intubation in the NC group (0.6% vs 6.3%, $P<.001$) and less need for chest compression in the NC group (1.65% vs 8.28%, $P<.001$) compared to the face mask group.[7] In 2014, Paz and colleagues, in a retrospective review of their experience in a single center using RAM NC for neonatal resuscitation in the delivery room, reported successful use in preterm and term newborns. Gestational age ranged from 23 to 41 weeks and BW ranged from 270 to 4675 g in this study.[8] In another study, Biniwale and colleagues reported a significant decrease in delivery room intubation rate, chest compressions, epinephrine administration, and the need for subsequent IMV in the NICU with the early start of nasal intermittent positive pressure ventilation (NIPPV) using RAM NC in the delivery room compared to positive pressure ventilation or nasal continuous positive airway pressure (NCPAP) applied using a face mask.[9] In a comparative study using RAM NC, Hudson nasal prongs, and nasal mask as interface, Sharma and colleagues showed that measured CPAP levels at the level of the hypopharynx in 90 preterm infants were low with all 3 of these nasal interfaces with nasal mask delivering pressure close to set NCPAP pressure. However, the difference between set versus measured pressure at the level of the hypopharynx ranged between 0.6 and 0.7 cm H_2O.[10] If one is using a nasal interface such as RAM NC or binasal prongs use of 1 cm H_2O higher than the usual CPAP pressure will deliver the pressure intended by the provider. In summary, based on evidence, the use of a simple nasal interface, such as RAM NC and NIPPV mode, in the delivery room for neonates with respiratory distress needing PPV results in less need for intubation, chest compressions, epinephrine use, and IMV after admission to the NICU.

RESPIRATORY SUPPORT IN THE NEWBORN INTENSIVE CARE UNIT

NIV modes: Several modes of NIV have been studied in neonates needing respiratory support (**Table 1**). These modes include NCPAP, sigh positive airway pressure (Si-PAP) or bilevel positive airway pressure (Bi-PAP) or duo positive airway pressure (Duo-PAP), NIPPV, high-flow nasal cannula (HFNC), nasal high-frequency oscillatory ventilation (NHFOV), nasal high-frequency jet ventilation (NHFJV), and NIV neurally adjusted ventilatory assist (NIV-NAVA). Delivery of NIV modes requires a source of gas flow, a resister to generate pressure at the level of the patient's nasal interface, and a nasal interface, such as a face mask, binasal prongs, binasal cannula, or nasopharyngeal prongs. Bilevel NIV modes such as Si-PAP or Bi-PAP are often used interchangeably with NIPPV. NIPPV is truly not just a "bilevel" NIV mode since the pressures used are much higher than "bilevel" NIV modes. When reviewing studies, one must pay careful attention to the exact mode that was used in the studies.

Nasal Continuous Positive Airway Pressure

NCPAP involves applying pressure to the airway of a spontaneously breathing newborn and works by maintaining functional residual capacity (FRC) and decreasing upper airway resistance. NCPAP may be delivered using bubble CPAP (bCPAP) with a constant flow or using variable flows using Si-PAP (Infant Flow SiPAP by Vyaire Medical) or Bi-PAP devices or using a conventional ventilator. Initial studies suggested that with oscillations of around 2 to 3 cm H_2O amplitude, bCPAP may work as a high-frequency ventilator to improve ventilation.[11] The investigators suggested that chest vibrations produced during bCPAP may offer an inexpensive option to improve gas exchange.

Recently, the Cochrane Database of Systematic Reviews included 15 RCTs involving 1437 preterm infants comparing bCPAP versus ventilator or infant flow-generated CPAP. The investigators concluded that there is a low level of certainty about the effects of bCPAP versus other pressure sources, such as ventilators or infant flow driver–generated CPAP on the risk of treatment failure and most associated morbidity and mortality for preterm infants.[12] The optimal starting pressure for NCPAP is not well established. Clinicians have recommended CPAP between 5 and 8 cm H_2O. Rarely, a CPAP of 10 cm H_2O or higher is used due to the adverse effects of high distending pressure on cardiac hemodynamics, causing a decrease in venous return as well as risks of air leaks. A recent study by Mukerji and colleagues used high CPAP pressures between 9 and 14 cm H_2O for a short duration and compared with NIPPV in a crossover design. They found no adverse outcomes with the use of high CPAP such as changes in cardiac output or work of breathing when compared to equivalent mean airway pressures (MAPs) used with NIPPV.[13]

NCPAP is beneficial but fails in more than 50% of very preterm infants.[14] Eight RCTs published between 2007 and 2013 from various places around the world showed failures with NCPAP within 5 days from birth, ranging from 33% to 52% (**Fig. 1**).[15–22] In addition, despite a substantial increase in the use of NCPAP, there was no decrease in BPD or improvement in lung function at 8 years of age.[23] This has led to the use of bilevel NIV modes and synchronized or non-synchronized NIPPV modes to decrease the need for intubation or reintubations and improve pulmonary outcomes.

Table 1
Noninvasive ventilation modes

	Flow Pattern	Typical Settings	Comments	Benefits	Risks
Nasal CPAP					
1. Bubble CPAP 2. Biphasic CPAP 3. Ventilator-generated CPAP	1. Continuous 2. Variable 3. Continuous	CPAP 5–8 cm H_2O	Clinical studies have shown no difference in short-term or long-term pulmonary outcomes between these 3 modes of NCPAP.	Improves V/Q mismatch and oxygenation Improves work of breathing Prevents atelectasis Less work of breathing	Nasal trauma Air leaks Gastric distention
Biphasic CPAP modes					
Biphasic modes: Si-PAP/Bi-PAP/Duo-PAP	Variable	PIP 10–15 cm H_2O PEEP 5–6 cm H_2O IT 0.6 s	Mimics CPAP; Delta pressure is low and failure rates needing IMV are similar to NCPAP; Needs high flow rates, longer IT, and maximum PIP is 10–15 cmH_2O	Same as CPAP Additional benefit to prevent apneas with variable pressures	Same as CPAP
NIPPV: Mimics IMV without an endotracheal tube					
Ventilator-generated sNIPPV	Variable	PIP 20–30 cm H_2O PEEP 5–8 cm H_2O	No limit on maximum PIP; Synchronization using Graseby capsule, Flow sensor or NAVA catheter	Benefits of CPAP Decrease need for mechanical ventilation	Same as CPAP
Ventilator Generated nsNIPPV	Variable		No limit on maximum PIP		
High-flow nasal cannula					
HFNC	Continuous	Flow rate 2–8 l pm	Pressure is neither measured nor controlled by the care provider, and hypopharyngeal Fio_2 varies depending on the patient's spontaneous breathing rate	Easier for nursing and parents Similar to CPAP Less gastric distention	Unmonitored pressures and may be high or ineffective

Nasal High-frequency ventilation					
Nasal HFOV	Continuous	See **Table 2**	Used as a primary mode or following extubation from IMV	Decrease apneas Increase CO_2 clearance	Limited data on safety and efficacy
Nasal HFJV	Variable	See **Table 2**	Limited data; Used in combination with NIPPV		
Synchronized NIPPV using a NAVA catheter					
NIV-NAVA	Variable	See **Table 3**.	Synchronization done using NAVA catheter	Improves patient ventilator synchrony Improves patient comfort Decreases pressures required	Limited efficacy Limited in extremely preterm infants due to immature respiratory control

Abbreviations: Bi-PAP, bilevel positive airway pressure; CPAP, continuous positive airway pressure; Duo-PAP, duo positive airway pressure; HFJV, high-frequency jet ventilation; HFNC, high-flow nasal cannula; HFOV, high-frequency oscillatory ventilation; IMV, invasive mechanical ventilation; IT, inspiratory time; NAVA, neurally adjusted ventilatory assist; NCPAP, nasal continuous positive airway pressure; NIPPV, nasal intermittent positive pressure ventilation; NIV-NAVA, noninvasive neurally adjusted ventilatory assist; nsNIPPV, nonsynchronized nasal intermittent positive pressure ventilation; PEEP, positive end-expiratory pressure; PIP, peak inspiratory pressure; Si-PAP, sigh positive airway pressure; sNIPPV, synchronized nasal intermittent positive pressure ventilation; V/Q, ventilation-perfusion.

NCPAP in the Delivery Room & Early Failures (Early MV [eMV] in the 1st 5 days) 2008-2013 (8 RCTs)

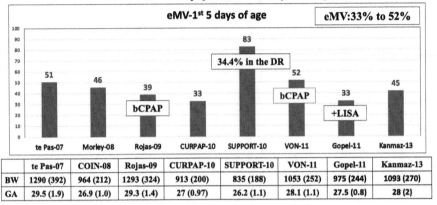

	te Pas-07	COIN-08	Rojas-09	CURPAP-10	SUPPORT-10	VON-11	Gopel-11	Kanmaz-13
BW	1290 (392)	964 (212)	1293 (324)	913 (200)	835 (188)	1053 (252)	975 (244)	1093 (270)
GA	29.5 (1.9)	26.9 (1.0)	29.3 (1.4)	27 (0.97)	26.2 (1.1)	28.1 (1.1)	27.5 (0.8)	28 (2)

Fig. 1. Nasal continuous positive airway pressure in the delivery room and failures needing mechanical ventilation within 5 days of birth. bCPAP, bubble continuous positive airway pressure; DR, delivery room; eMV, early mechanical ventilation; GA, gestational age; LISA, less invasive surfactant administration.

Synchronized Intermittent Positive Airway Pressure or Bilevel Positive Airway Pressure or Duo Positive Airway Pressure

These devices use 2 different flow rates to generate biphasic modalities with high pressure (peak inspiratory pressure [PIP]) and low pressure (positive end-expiratory pressure [PEEP]). They also provide a backup rate. A Si-PAP device uses 2 different channels to deliver the gases. The direction of gas flow changes with the infant's breathing patterns while maintaining a relatively constant CPAP throughout the breathing cycle. Furthermore, when the patient begins to exhale, the gas flow is diverted to the exhalation tube, thus minimizing expiratory resistance and work of breathing. This mechanism to deliver gas flow is known as fluidic flip and is based on the Coanda effect, that is, a stream of gas coming out from a nozzle that tends to follow a nearby curved surface with the least resistance. The CPAP generator relies on the newborn's breathing effort to trigger the fluidic flip. Bi-PAP provides biphasic CPAPs and a backup rate similar to Si-PAP. Despite these theoretic advantages of the Coanda effect, clinical trials have not shown any difference in failure rates when compared to conventional ventilator-delivered CPAP.[24] Typical pressure settings used with Si-PAP or Bi-PAP are 10 to 12/6 cm H_2O with a delta pressure of 4 to 6 cm H_2O. In patients with high partial pressure of carbon dioxide (Pco_2), it is not possible to improve ventilation with such a low delta pressure since delta pressure is the one that controls delivered tidal volume. RCTs comparing Si-PAP or Bi-PAP with NCPAP have shown no difference between these 3 modes of NIV. Kirpalani and colleagues published the largest trial in 1009 extremely low-BW infants comparing bilevel NIV versus NCPAP.[25] Although the title of this study is "A Trial Comparing NIV Strategies in Preterm Infants," this multicenter, multinational trial truly was a study comparing Si-PAP versus NCPAP since 52% of the participating centers used a Si-PAP device to deliver "NIPPV." Furthermore, maximum PIP was limited to 18 cm H_2O even when using a conventional ventilator to deliver "NIPPV" due to concerns for gastrointestinal perforation.[26] In another RCT involving 540 preterm infants less than 30 weeks of GA, comparing Bi-PAP versus NCPAP showed failure rates needing reintubation were similar (21% vs 20%) between the 2 groups. There was no difference in BPD between the 2 modes.[27] In a systematic review and meta-analysis of 14 trials involving 1392 subjects, Bharadwaj and colleagues found no difference in BPD or mortality between bCPAP, infant flow–driven CPAP, and ventilator-generated CPAP. Interestingly, they found a higher rate of nasal injuries in the bCPAP group (risk ratio [RR] 2.04, 95% confidence interval [CI] 1.33, 3.14).[28] Sadeghnia and colleagues from Iran, in a small RCT comparing Bi-PAP versus Si-PAP in 74 preterm infants, found no difference in BPD or death between these 2 bilevel modes.[29] In summary, there are no differences in failure rates needing intubation, BPD, or death between NCPAP, Si-PAP, or Bi-PAP. Preterm infants failing NCPAP will likely fail Bi-PAP or Si-PAP, and therefore, other modes of NIV, such as NIPPV or NHFV, should be used in these patients failing NCPAP or bilevel CPAP modes.

Nasal Intermittent Positive Pressure Ventilation

NIPPV truly mimics IMV, except without the need for an endotracheal tube. Typical settings used when initiating NIPPV are PIP/PEEP of 20/6 cm H_2O, inspiratory time (IT) of 0.5 seconds, and a rate of 40 bpm. This provides a delta pressure of 14 cm H_2O which helps with improving ventilation in patients with hypercarbia. Several mechanisms have been proposed regarding the effects of NIPPV. They are (1) pharyngeal dilation with a decrease in upper airway resistance, (2) activation of the Head's paradoxical reflex, (3) increase in FRC, (4) increase in tidal volume and minute volume, (5) alveolar recruitment due to higher MAP, (6) reduction in chest wall distortion, (7) increase in respiratory drive, and (8) decrease in work of breathing. Synchronized NIPPV (sNIPPV) as well as non-synchronized (nsNIPPV) have been studied in clinical trials. Synchronization with the patient's spontaneous inspiratory effort is done using a Graseby capsule, flow synchronization, or neurally adjusted ventilatory assist (NAVA). No studies compare sNIPPV versus nsNIPPV.

A large number of RCTs comparing NCPAP versus NIPPV modes and 3 systematic reviews on the comparison of NCPAP with NIPPV have been published. Ten RCTs comparing NCPAP versus NIPPV demonstrated that failure rates with NIPPV needing intubation or reintubation were significantly lower with NIPPV (5% to 25%) (**Fig. 2**).[30–39] Ferguson and colleagues, in a systematic review and meta-analysis of 9 RCTs, comparing NCPAP versus sNIPPV or nsNIPPV and mixed mode including Si-PAP and NIPPV concluded that both sNIPPV and nsNIPPV modes are superior to NCPAP in preventing extubation failures, with a number needed to treat of 8 (95% CI 2,5).[40] They concluded that preterm infants should be extubated to NIV mode of respiratory support, and caffeine should be used routinely. A meta-analysis, including postextubation support by any mode of NIPPV or Bi-PAP, demonstrated superiority over NCPAP in preventing extubation failures. In a 2017 Cochrane systematic review and meta-analysis from 10 RCTs involving 1061 patients, Lemyre and colleagues concluded that early NIPPV does appear superior to NCPAP alone for decreasing respiratory failure and the need for intubation and IMV among preterm infants with RDS (RR 0.65, 95% CI 0.51, 0.82, *P*=.0004).[40] They also evaluated the devices used to deliver NIV and synchronized NIPPV. Ventilator-delivered NIPPV had the lowest failure rates with a number needed to benefit (NNTB) of 13 (95% CI 7, 50) and nsNIPPV also decreased extubation failures significantly (RR 0.60, 95% CI 0.44, 0.83). In 2020, 2 systematic reviews and network meta-analyses have been published. In the first review, the use of NIPPV as a primary mode of support in preterm infants with RDS was reported including, 35 studies with 4078 patients. The authors concluded that the most effective NIV mode for primary respiratory support in preterm infants with RDS was NIPPV. The need for IMV with NIPPV was significantly lower when compared to NCPAP (RR

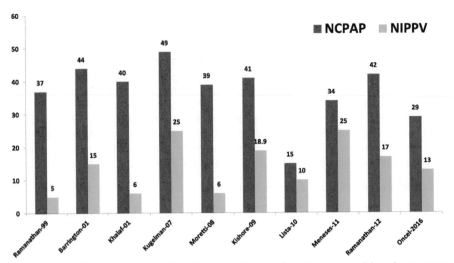

Fig. 2. Ten randomized controlled trials comparing nasal continuous positive airway pressure versus nasal intermittent positive pressure ventilation between 1999 and 2016: Failures needing invasive mechanical ventilation. NCPAP, nasal continuous positive airway pressure; NIPPV, nasal intermittent positive pressure ventilation.

0.60, 95% CI 0.44, 077). NIPPV resulted in a lesser incidence of BPD or mortality when compared to NCPAP (RR o.74, 95% CI 0.52, 0,98).[41]

The same authors also reported results from 33 RCTs involving 3899 subjects regarding the use of NIV modes for post-extubation respiratory support in preterm infants with RDS. In this systematic review and network meta-analysis, sNIPPV was found to be the most effective, and continuous flow CPAP the least effective modality for preventing respiratory failure in preterm neonates. nsNIPPV also resulted in lesser reintubation compared to variable flow CPAP (RR 0.61, 95% CI 0.36, 0.97) and HFNC (RR 0.49, 95% CI 0.27, 0.80).[42] These results are consistent with Lemyre and colleagues' findings. To date, no studies have compared sNIPPV versus nsNIPPV in a pairwise manner assessing the clinical outcomes. Both sNIPPV and nsNIPPV are better than NCPAP or Bi-PAP/Si-PAP in decreasing the need for IMV. In a recent retrospective cohort study involving 156 preterm infants, NIPPV as a rescue therapy reduced the need for IMV in infants who failed NCPAP and was associated with better clinical outcomes.[43] In a randomized crossover trial, the use of sNIPPV when compared to NHOV resulted in fewer desaturation episodes and lower Fio_2 exposure.[44] In summary, among all the biphasic (Si-PAP or Bi-PAP) or NIPPV modes for respiratory support, sNIPPV, as well as nsNIPPV, is superior when used as a primary mode or following a period of IMV in improving pulmonary outcomes. Settings for application of NIPPV for initiation, weaning phase, and chronic phase are shown in **Table 2**. One has to use higher pressures to overcome the resistance of the nasal interfaces, compensate for leaks, and have a longer IT to match the longer time constants during NIV mode. With the availability of NIV Plus software in Medtronic PB 980 ventilator, care providers can optimize settings based on actual pressures measured at the tip of the nasal interfaces and with good leak compensation.[45] In chronic patients with severe BPD, the use of NIPPV with higher PIP/PEEP may lead to sustained improvement.[46] Additionally, NIPPV is found to be beneficial in avoiding tracheostomies for patients with significant laryngotracheomalacia, optimizing the time of surgery in patients with subglottic stenosis and stabilizing airway after aryepiglottoplasty.[47]

Table 2
Suggested nasal intermittent positive pressure ventilation settings for use as a primary mode or following extubation from invasive mechanical ventilation

	Initial Settings	Weaning Phase	Chronic Phase
PIP (cm H_2O)	20, may increase up to 30 cm H_2O	12–15, wean by 2 cm H_2O every 6 h	30–35
PEEP (cm H_2O)	6, may increase up to 8 cm H_2O	≤ 5	8–10
IT (s)	0.5	0.5	0.5
Rate (bpm)	40	20	30–40

Abbreviations: bpm, beats per minute; IT, inspiratory time; PEEP, positive end-expiratory pressure; PIP, peak inspiratory pressure.

Nasal interfaces during nasal continuous positive airway pressure/noninvasive ventilation

Multiple types of nasal interfaces have been used to provide NIV support in newborns. These include Hudson prongs, INCA prongs, Fisher-Packer nasal prongs/mask, Argyle prongs, and RAM NC. The risk of nasal septal or columellar injuries is common with binasal prongs.[48] Nasal injuries were seen in 13.2% within 7 days of NCPAP. Columellar necrosis was seen in 5.5% of patients as early as 10 days after NCPAP. Careful attention to the nostrils in patients on NIV support by the nursing, respiratory, and clinical care team is extremely important. Careful documentation of prong position and any evidence of redness or ulceration are important to prevent the worsening of nasal injuries. Alternating binasal prongs with nasal masks have also been utilized to decrease the risk of nasal injuries.[49] Using nasal masks alone as compared to binasal prongs has also been shown to decrease nasal injury as well as CPAP failure.[50] Application of a neoseal or Cannulaide or DuoDERM between the nostrils and nasal interfaces has also been recommended.

The authors designed a simple nasal interface called RAM NC more than 10 years ago and several RCTs have shown that RAM NC use for NIV support has been shown to result in significantly fewer nasal injuries and with equal efficiency and safety. Three RCTs have been published evaluating RAM NC versus binasal prongs to deliver NIPPV. In the RCT from Israel by Hochwald and colleagues, NIPPV using RAM NC resulted in similar efficacy but with significantly decreased rates of moderate to severe nasal injuries (5% vs 17%) when compared to binasal prongs and/or nasal masks.[51] In an RCT from India, Maram and colleagues compared RAM NC with Hudson prongs to deliver NCPAP and concluded that RAM NC compared to Hudson prongs decreased nasal injury (5.4% vs 26.4%) without increasing the need for IMV.[52] In another RCT from a low-income and middle-income country, Samim and colleagues compared RAM NC versus short binasal prongs for NCPAP in 254 preterm infants between 28 and 34 weeks GA and found the incidence of moderate to severe nasal injury was significantly lower in the group randomized to RAM NC (2.4% vs 8.7%, $P \leq .028$) and mean duration of CPAP was also significantly shorter (52 hours vs 65 hours, $P = .017$) when compared to short binasal prongs.[53] RAM NC can be used to deliver NCPAP and NIPPV in the delivery room, and all modes of NIV, including NIPPV, NHFOV, NHFJV, and NIV-NAVA, in the NICU. In summary, based on evidence, the use of sNIPPV or nsNIPPV as a primary mode or following extubation from IMV to support preterm infants with RDS has been shown to be superior to NCPAP, Bi-PAP, or Si-PAP. Patient-friendly nasal interface like RAM NC has also been shown to effective and safe in providing all modes of NIV with a significant decrease in nasal injuries.

Noninvasive Neurally Adjusted Ventilatory Assist

NIV-NAVA is one of the modes that can provide synchronized NIV in infants. Synchronization is achieved by the signal-capturing electrical activity of the diaphragm (Edi) via electrodes attached to the nasogastric tube. Edi catheter is connected to the ventilator, which detects diaphragmatic electric activity and assists in providing proportional breaths. Edi peak is the highest Edi value during the breath and corresponds to the amount of electric activity needed to generate adequate tidal volume and is representative of diaphragmatic workload. Edi min is the lowest value that represents the baseline resting of the diaphragm that prevents derecruitment. The mechanism of NIV-NAVA is to provide proportionate breaths while maintaining Edi peak levels between 5 and 15 μV and Edi min levels between 2 and 4 μV while synchronizing with diaphragmatic contractions. The level of support provided is referred to as the NAVA level. Parameters that need to be set after placing infants on NIV-NAVA ventilation include PEEP, fraction of inspired oxygen, NAVA level, apnea time, which is the backup rate set for apnea prevention, and peak pressure limit. Edi trigger is typically set at 0.5 μV, and cycling off is typically at 70% of Edi.[54] NAVA levels are adjusted for work of breathing and Edi peak, whereas PEEP is adjusted for Edi min levels (**Table 3**).

Clinical studies on NIV-NAVA have shown benefits with patient synchrony,[55,56] improvement in oxygen requirement,[56–58] and a decrease in reintubation rates.[58,59] Currently, a large multicenter RCT (NCT05446272) is underway to assess the outcomes of infants placed on NIV-NAVA compared with NIPPV. The main advantage of NIV-NAVA is the ability to synchronize breaths, which is potentially beneficial for preterm infants to decrease the risk of long-term complications. The limitations of this mode include a lack of robust clinical studies to prove its utility, especially for long-term benefits, and the need for the use of a Servo ventilator, which may not be readily available at most institutions.

Table 3
Suggested settings for noninvasive neurally adjusted ventilatory assist

	Initial Settings	Maximum	Adjust by	Minimum
NAVA level	1 cm H_2O/μV	4 cm H_2O/μV	0.1–0.2 cm H_2O/μV	0.5 cm H_2O/μV
Edi max between 5–15 μV	For Edi max >20 μV, increase NAVA level; If Edi max is < 5, decrease NAVA level; NAVA levels in NIV-NAVA are usually **lower** than in invasive NAVA; Usual NAVA level is 0.5–1.			
PEEP, cm H2O	6	8–10	1	5
Edi min (2–4 μV) & PEEP adjustments	If Edi min is constantly above 1, increase PEEP; If Edi min is too low, decrease PEEP			
Edi trigger	0.5 μV	2 μV	Adjust as needed	
Backup pressure control above PEEP	15 cm H_2O	30–35 cm H_2O	1–2 cm H_2O	Per NIPPV
Rate	30/min	Per NIPPV	Per NIPPV	Per NIPPV
Inspiratory time	0.5 s	-	-	-
Trigger sensitivity	1–2	-	-	-
High-pressure alarm	40 cm H_2O	-	-	-

Abbreviations: Edi, electrical activity of the diaphragm; NAVA, neurally adjusted ventilatory assist; NIPPV, nasal intermittent positive pressure ventilation; NIV-NAVA, noninvasive neurally adjusted ventilatory assist; PEEP, positive end-expiratory pressure.

Nasal High-Frequency Ventilation

High-frequency ventilation has been most often used in NICU, typically in the form of rescue mode for clinical deterioration of infants with conventional ventilation. NHFOV has been the most widely studied. The mechanism of action of NHFOV relates to providing continuous positive pressure to distend the lungs with added oscillations to aid the gas exchange. The biggest advantage of NHFOV over CPAP is that clinicians can administer much higher MAPs for lung recruitment while avoiding gas trapping due to added oscillations. Tidal volume oscillations are impacted by IT, amplitude, and frequency adjusted on the oscillator. Increasing IT and amplitude may deliver a larger tidal volume which, could also be achieved by decreasing frequency. Larger size of nasal prongs used to provide noninvasive support may help better delivery of volume.[60] Nasal masks may not be able to provide similar volumes due to leaks, and clinicians may need to consider using higher settings to achieve optimized ventilation.[61]

The initial pilot study performed using a nasal high-frequency percussive ventilator improved oxygenation of infants diagnosed with transient tachypnea of the newborn in 40 patients.[62] Several studies performed using NHFOV showed its beneficial effects in avoiding reintubation and increased carbon dioxide clearance. Systematic review and meta-analysis performed using pooled data from the individual studies involving 570 infants revealed that NHFOV significantly reduced reintubation rates compared to CPAP.[63] Another meta-analysis comparing NHFOV to NIPPV in 1138 infants showed its potential to decrease reintubation without risking complications, although the long-term outcomes, including BPD, were not different between the groups.[64]

Suggested settings for NHFOV are described in **Table 4**. Settings are adjusted based on oxygenation, ventilation, chest expansion, as well as patient's comfort status.

Table 4
Suggested nasal high-frequency ventilation settings

Ventilator	Suggested Initial HFV Settings	Suggested Initial IMV Settings
3100A	Frequency: 8–10 Hz I:E ratio: 1:2 or 1:1 MAP (P_{aw}): Similar to IMV or CPAP Amp/ Delta P: 2 x MAP	No conventional breaths
VDR4 or Bronchotron	Frequency: 5–8 Hz I:E ratio: 1:1 MAP: Similar to IMV or CPAP	Optional NIPPV breaths Frequency 6–20 bpm PIP as needed to move chest
Drager VN500 or Babylog 8000	Frequency: 6–10 Hz Amp/Delta P: 2 x MAP I:E ratio: 1:1 MAP: Similar to IMV or CPAP	Optional NIPPV breaths Frequency 6–20 bpm PIP: 15–20 above MAP (P_{aw}) as needed to move chest
Leoni Plus/Stephanie/ Sophie	Variable I:E ratio	Same as mentioned earlier
HFJV—LifePulse jet ventilator	Frequency: 4 Hz Valve on time: 0.03 s	NIPPV breaths—PIP/PEEP 20–30/6–10 cm H_2O, NIPPV rate 40 bpm, IT 0.5 s

Abbreviations: bpm, beats per minute; CPAP, continuous positive airway pressure; HFV, high-frequency ventilation; I:E, inspiratory to expiratory time; IMV, invasive mechanical ventilation; IT, inspiratory time; MAP, mean airway pressure; NIPPV, nasal intermittent positive pressure ventilation; Paw, mean airway pressure.

Nasal high-frequency jet ventilation (NFHJV) has only been studied in the form of its successful use in a case series published by the authors' institution. Its use in conjunction with NIPPV showed improvement in pulmonary status in extremely preterm infants to avoid reintubation in 81% of the patients. The majority of these infants received invasive jet ventilation followed by extubation to NHFJV or as rescue therapy when NIPPV failed. Typical settings included higher PEEP by 1 to 3 cm H_2O and higher PIP by 2 to 10 cm H_2O. Unlike the invasive jet ventilation, during NHFJV full support of pressures and rates were provided by conventional ventilator delivering NIPPV.[65] Further studies are needed before its routine use in clinical practice.

High-Flow Nasal Cannula

Heated, humidified HFNC has been used as a form of NIV mode in preterm infants. Although the physiologic effects of HFNC are still under investigation, their mechanisms of action include the generation of PEEP, reduction of the work of breathing, and clearance of the nasopharyngeal dead space, while providing optimal gas conditioning. However, a major issue with the HFNC system is that the delivered pressure is neither measured nor controlled by the care provider. In addition, the hypopharyngeal concentration of inspired oxygen varies with the spontaneous breathing rate of the patients. Taha and colleagues reported the results from a large retrospective data analysis from the Alere Neonatal Database for extremely low-BW infants (<1000 g) at birth who received HFNC or NCPAP. A total of 2487 infants (941 CPAP group, 333 HFNC group, and 1546 HFNC ± CPAP group) were included in this study. The primary outcome of BPD or death was significantly higher in the HFNC group (56.8%) compared with the CPAP group (50.4%, $P < .05$). Similarly, adjusted odds of developing BPD or death were greater in the HFNC ± CPAP group compared with the CPAP group (odds ratio 1.085, 95% CI 1.035–1.137, $P = .001$). The days on IMV, postnatal steroid use, days to room air, days to initiate or reach full oral feeds, and length of hospitalization were significantly higher in the HFNC and HFNC ± CPAP groups compared with the CPAP group.[66] Roberts and colleagues compared HFNC versus NCPAP for primary respiratory support in 564 preterm infants greater than 28 weeks GA in a multinational RCT (HIPSTER [A multicentre, randomised controlled, non-inferiority trial, comparing high flow therapy with nasal continuous positive airway pressure as primary support for preterm infants with respiratory distress] trial). Treatment failure within 72 hours of randomization was 25.5% in the HFNC group versus 13.3% in the CPAP group ($P < .001$).[67] In another RCT in preterm infants (>28 weeks GA, mean BW 1632 g vs 1642 g) with RDS, comparing HFNC [5–7 lpm] versus NCPAP at 5 cm H_2O for primary respiratory support, the need for IMV within 72 hours was significantly higher in the HFNC group (26.3% vs 7.9%, $P \leq .0001$). This study was stopped after a planned interim analysis (272 out of 460 patients were enrolled).[68] In a recent Cochrane database systematic review of nasal highflow (nHF) therapy for primary respiratory support in preterm infants, 13 studies involving 2540 infants were included. The investigators concluded that nHF use for primary respiratory support in preterm infants of greater than 28 weeks GA results in an increase in treatment failure within 72 hours of study entry but no significant differences in any morbidities, and there is a lack of evidence in infants less than 28 weeks for the use nHF.[69] In an RCT comparing HFNC (6–8 lpm flow) versus NCPAP (6–8 cm H_2O) in 754 preterm infants greater than 31 weeks GA (mean GA 36.9 weeks, mean BW 2909 g) from 9 nontertiary special care nurseries in Australia for early respiratory support, HFNC therapy was associated significantly higher rate of treatment failures (20.5% vs 10.2%).[70] Uchiyama and colleagues compared HFNC with NCPAP or NIPPV after extubation from IMV in an RCT from 6 NICUs in Japan (n = 372; mean

GA weeks 28.4 vs 28.2 weeks, mean BW 1129 g vs 1070 g). They used flow rates of 2 to 8 lpm in the HFNC group and 4 to 5 cm H_2O in the NCPAP group. HFNC resulted in significantly higher failure rates within 72 hours, as well as within 7 days (31% vs 16%) after extubation.[71] In summary, HFNC is not patient friendly based on studies; pressure and oxygen delivery are variable and unpredictable and may result in prolonged exposure to pressure or oxygen. HFNC may be used postextubation in babies greater than 1250 g. It may be safer to use NCPAP or NIPPV where care providers can control the pressure.

SUMMARY

NIPPV, when used as a primary mode or following a period of IMV, decreases the need for intubation, mechanical ventilation, and BPD. A limited number of RCTs have shown a decrease in death or BPD with NIPPV. NIPPV is safe, feasible, effective, and easy to implement. Failures are similar to NCPAP versus Bi-PAP/Si-PAP or DuoPAP. NHFV may be used as a rescue mode when NIPPV fails. NIV-NAVA is a promising mode awaiting larger clinical trials. Future RCTs are needed to compare sNIPPV versus nsNIPPV in preterm infants with respiratory distress.

CLINICS CARE POINTS

- Noninvasive mechanical ventilation requires careful bedside monitoring by nursing and respiratory care practitioners to make sure that there is a gap between nasal interface and the columella part of the nares to minimize the risk of nasal injuries.

- Abdominal distention due to gas going through the lower esophageal sphincter is a major issue, and frequent aspiration of gas before feedings is needed to decrease feeding intolerance.

- It is important to have at least 20% to 30% leak around the nasal interfaces to minimize the risk of nasal injuries and to decrease the expiratory resistance and work of breathing, by allowing patients to exhale around the nasal interfaces.

DISCLOSURE

Dr R. Ramanathan has a joint patent with Neotech Products, Inc, and receives royalties. Dr R. Ramanathan donates all honorarium payments to charities around the world to help mothers, children, and newborns. Dr M. Biniwale has nothing to disclose regarding this work.

REFERENCES

1. Stoll BJ, Hansen NI, Bell EF, et al. Trends in care practices, morbidity, and mortality of extremely preterm neonates, 1993-2012. JAMA 2015;314(10):1039–51.
2. Bohrer B, Silveira RC, Neto EC, et al. Mechanical ventilation of newborns infant changes in plasma pro- and anti-inflammatory cytokines. J Pediatr 2010;156(1):16–9.
3. Bose CL, Laughon MM, Allred EN, et al. Systemic inflammation associated with mechanical ventilation among extremely preterm infants. Cytokine 2013;61(1):315–22.
4. Machumpurath S, O'Currain E, Dawson JA, et al. Interfaces for non-invasive neonatal resuscitation in the delivery room: a systematic review and meta-analysis. Resuscitation 2020;156:244–50.

5. Schmölzer GM, Dawson JA, Kamlin CO, et al. Airway obstruction and gas leak during mask ventilation of preterm infants in the delivery room. Arch Dis Child Fetal Neonatal Ed 2011;96(4):F254–7.

6. Kuypers KLAM, Lamberska T, Martherus T, et al. The effect of a face mask for respiratory support on breathing in preterm infants at birth. Resuscitation 2019;144: 178–84.

7. Capasso L, Capasso A, Raimondi F, et al. A randomized trial comparing oxygen delivery on intermittent positive pressure with nasal cannulae versus facial mask in neonatal primary resuscitation. Acta Paediatr. Feb 2005;94(2):197–200.

8. Paz P, Ramanathan R, Hernandez R, et al. Neonatal resuscitation using a nasal cannula: a single-center experience. Am J Perinatol 2014;31(12):1031–6.

9. Biniwale M, Wertheimer F. Decrease in delivery room intubation rates after use of nasal intermittent positive pressure ventilation in the delivery room for resuscitation of very low birth weight infants. Resuscitation 2017;116:33–8.

10. Sharma D, Murki S, Maram S, et al. Comparison of delivered distending pressures in the oropharynx in preterm infants on bubble CPAP and three different nasal interfaces. Pediatr Pulmonol 2020;55(7):1631–9.

11. Lee KS, Dunn MS, Fenwick M, et al. A comparison of underwater bubble continuous positive airway pressure with ventilator-derived continuous positive airway pressure in premature neonates ready for extubation. Biol Neonate 1998;73(2): 69–75.

12. Prakash R, De Paoli AG, Davis PG, et al. Bubble devices versus other pressure sources for nasal continuous positive airway pressure in preterm infants. Cochrane Database Syst Rev 2023;3(3):CD015130.

13. Mukerji A, Abdul Wahab MG, Razak A, et al. High CPAP vs. NIPPV in preterm neonates - a physiological cross-over study. J Perinatol 2021;41(7):1690–6.

14. Fischer HS, Bührer C. Avoiding endotracheal ventilation to prevent bronchopulmonary dysplasia: a meta-analysis. Pediatrics 2013;132(5):e1351–60.

15. te Pas AB, Walther FJ. A randomized, controlled trial of delivery-room respiratory management in very preterm infants. Pediatrics 2007;120(2):322–9.

16. Morley CJ, Davis PG, Doyle LW, et al. Nasal CPAP or intubation at birth for very preterm infants. N Engl J Med 2008;358(7):700–8.

17. Rojas MA, Lozano JM, Rojas MX, et al. Very early surfactant without mandatory ventilation in premature infants treated with early continuous positive airway pressure: a randomized, controlled trial. Pediatrics 2009;123(1):137–42.

18. Sandri F, Plavka R, Ancora G, et al. Prophylactic or early selective surfactant combined with nCPAP in very preterm infants. Pediatrics 2010;125(6):e1402–9.

19. Finer NN, Carlo WA, Walsh MC, et al. Early CPAP versus surfactant in extremely preterm infants. N Engl J Med 2010;362(21):1970–9.

20. Dunn MS, Kaempf J, de Klerk A, et al. A randomized trial comparing 3 approaches to the initial respiratory management of preterm neonates. Pediatrics 2011;128(5):e1069–76.

21. Göpel W, Kribs A, Ziegler A, et al. Avoidance of mechanical ventilation by surfactant treatment of spontaneously breathing preterm infants (AMV): an open-label, randomised, controlled trial. Lancet 2011;378(9803):1627–34.

22. Kanmaz HG, Erdeve O, Canpolat FE, et al. Surfactant administration via a thin catheter during spontaneous breathing: randomized controlled trial. Pediatrics 2013;131(2):e502–9.

23. Doyle LW, Carse E, Adams AM, et al. Ventilation in extremely preterm infants and respiratory function at 8 Years. N Engl J Med 2017;377(4):329–37.

24. Stefanescu BM, Murphy WP, Hansell BJ, et al. A randomized, controlled trial comparing two different continuous positive airway pressure systems for the successful extubation of extremely low birth weight infants. Pediatrics 2003;112(5): 1031–8.
25. Kirpalani H, Millar D, Lemyre B, et al. A trial comparing noninvasive ventilation strategies in preterm infants. N Engl J Med 2013;369(7):611–20.
26. Garland JS, Nelson DB, Rice T, et al. Increased risk of gastrointestinal perforations in neonates mechanically ventilated with either face mask or nasal prongs. Pediatrics 1985;76(3):406–10.
27. Victor S, Roberts SA, Mitchell S, et al. Biphasic positive airway pressure or continuous positive airway pressure: a randomized trial. Pediatrics 2016;138(2).
28. Bharadwaj SK, Alonazi A, Banfield L, et al. Bubble versus other continuous positive airway pressure forms: a systematic review and meta-analysis. Arch Dis Child Fetal Neonatal Ed 2020;105(5):526–31.
29. Sadeghnia A, Danaei N, Barkatein B. A comparison of the effect of nasal bi-level positive airway pressure and sigh-positive airway pressure on the treatment of the preterm newborns weighing less than 1500 g affiliated with respiratory distress syndrome. Int J Prev Med 2016;7:21.
30. Friedlich P, Lecart C, Posen R, et al. A randomized trial of nasopharyngeal-synchronized intermittent mandatory ventilation versus nasopharyngeal continuous positive airway pressure in very low birth weight infants after extubation. J Perinatol 1999;19(6 Pt 1):413–8.
31. Barrington KJ, Bull D, Finer NN. Randomized trial of nasal synchronized intermittent mandatory ventilation compared with continuous positive airway pressure after extubation of very low birth weight infants. Pediatrics 2001;107(4):638–41.
32. Khalaf MN, Brodsky N, Hurley J, et al. A prospective randomized, controlled trial comparing synchronized nasal intermittent positive pressure ventilation versus nasal continuous positive airway pressure as modes of extubation. Pediatrics 2001;108(1):13–7.
33. Kugelman A, Feferkorn I, Riskin A, et al. Nasal intermittent mandatory ventilation versus nasal continuous positive airway pressure for respiratory distress syndrome: a randomized, controlled, prospective study. J Pediatr 2007;150(5): 521–6.
34. Moretti C, Giannini L, Fassi C, et al. Nasal flow-synchronized intermittent positive pressure ventilation to facilitate weaning in very low-birthweight infants: unmasked randomized controlled trial. Pediatr Int 2008;50(1):85–91.
35. Sai Sunil Kishore M, Dutta S, Kumar P. Early nasal intermittent positive pressure ventilation versus continuous positive airway pressure for respiratory distress syndrome. Acta Paediatr 2009;98(9):1412–5.
36. Lista G, Castoldi F, Fontana P, et al. Nasal continuous positive airway pressure (CPAP) versus bi-level nasal CPAP in preterm babies with respiratory distress syndrome: a randomised control trial. Arch Dis Child Fetal Neonatal Ed 2010; 95(2):F85–9.
37. Meneses J, Bhandari V, Alves JG, et al. Noninvasive ventilation for respiratory distress syndrome: a randomized controlled trial. Pediatrics 2011;127(2):300–7.
38. Ramanathan R, Sekar KC, Rasmussen M, et al. Nasal intermittent positive pressure ventilation after surfactant treatment for respiratory distress syndrome in preterm infants <30 weeks' gestation: a randomized, controlled trial. J Perinatol 2012;32(5):336–43.
39. Oncel MY, Arayici S, Uras N, et al. Nasal continuous positive airway pressure versus nasal intermittent positive-pressure ventilation within the minimally

invasive surfactant therapy approach in preterm infants: a randomised controlled trial. Arch Dis Child Fetal Neonatal Ed 2016;101(4):F323–8.

40. Ferguson KN, Roberts CT, Manley BJ, et al. Interventions to improve rates of successful extubation in preterm infants: a systematic review and meta-analysis. JAMA Pediatrb 2017;171(2):165–74.

41. Ramaswamy VV, More K, Roehr CC, et al. Efficacy of noninvasive respiratory support modes for primary respiratory support in preterm neonates with respiratory distress syndrome: systematic review and network meta-analysis. Pediatr Pulmonol 2020;55(11):2940–63.

42. Ramaswamy VV, Bandyopadhyay T, Nanda D, et al. Efficacy of noninvasive respiratory support modes as post-extubation respiratory support in preterm neonates: a systematic review and network meta-analysis. Pediatr Pulmonol 2020; 55(11):2924–39.

43. Ishigami AC, Meneses J, Alves JG, et al. Nasal intermittent positive pressure ventilation as a rescue therapy after nasal continuous positive airway pressure failure in infants with respiratory distress syndrome. J Perinatol 2023;43(3):311–6.

44. Atanasov S, Dippel C, Takoulegha D, et al. Fluctuations in oxygen saturation during synchronized nasal intermittent positive pressure ventilation and nasal high-frequency oscillatory ventilation in very low birth weight infants: a randomized crossover trial. Neonatology 2023;1–9.

45. Borg U, Aviano J, Ginani M, et al. Evaluation of common nasal cannulas in neonatal noninvasive ventilation (NIV) using a novel neonatal nasal model. Med Devices (Auckl) 2022;15:307–15.

46. Mann C, Bär W. Severe bronchopulmonary dysplasia improved by noninvasive positive pressure ventilation: a case report. J Med Case Rep 2011;5:435.

47. Wormald R, Naude A, Rowley H. Non-invasive ventilation in children with upper airway obstruction. Int J Pediatr Otorhinolaryngol 2009;73(4):551–4.

48. Jatana KR, Oplatek A, Stein M, et al. Effects of nasal continuous positive airway pressure and cannula use in the neonatal intensive care unit setting. Arch Otolaryngol Head Neck Surg 2010;136(3):287–91.

49. Gautam G, Gupta N, Sasidharan R, et al. Systematic rotation versus continuous application of 'nasal prongs' or 'nasal mask' in preterm infants on nCPAP: a randomized controlled trial. Eur J Pediatr 2023;182(6):2645–54.

50. Sardar S, Pal S, Ghosh M. A three-arm randomized, controlled trial of different nasal interfaces on the safety and efficacy of nasal intermittent positive-pressure ventilation in preterm newborns. Indian J Pediatr 2022;89(12): 1195–201.

51. Hochwald O, Riskin A, Borenstein-Levin L, et al. Cannula with long and narrow tubing vs short binasal prongs for noninvasive ventilation in preterm infants: noninferiority randomized clinical trial. JAMA Pediatr 2021;175(1):36–43.

52. Maram S, Murki S, Nayyar S, et al. RAM cannula with Cannulaide versus Hudson prongs for delivery of nasal continuous positive airway pressure in preterm infants: an RCT. Sci Rep 2021;11(1):23527.

53. Samim SK, Debata PK, Yadav A, et al. RAM cannula versus short binasal prongs for nasal continuous positive airway pressure delivery in preterm infants: a randomized, noninferiority trial from low-middle-income country. Eur J Pediatr 2022;181(12):4111–9.

54. Stein H, Beck J, Dunn M. Non-invasive ventilation with neurally adjusted ventilatory assist in newborns. Semin Fetal Neonatal Med 2016;21(3):154–61.

55. Lee J, Kim HS, Jung YH, et al. Non-invasive neurally adjusted ventilatory assist in preterm infants: a randomised phase II crossover trial. Arch Dis Child Fetal Neonatal Ed. Nov 2015;100(6):F507–13.

56. Gibu CK, Cheng PY, Ward RJ, et al. Feasibility and physiological effects of noninvasive neurally adjusted ventilatory assist in preterm infants. Pediatr Res 2017; 82(4):650–7.

57. Yagui AC, Meneses J, Zólio BA, et al. Nasal continuous positive airway pressure (NCPAP) or noninvasive neurally adjusted ventilatory assist (NIV-NAVA) for preterm infants with respiratory distress after birth: a randomized controlled trial. Pediatr Pulmonol 2019;54(11):1704–11.

58. Yagui AC, Gonçalves PA, Murakami SH, et al. Is noninvasive neurally adjusted ventilatory assistance (NIV-NAVA) an alternative to NCPAP in preventing extubation failure in preterm infants? J Matern Fetal Neonatal Med 2021;34(22):3756–60.

59. Lee BK, Shin SH, Jung YH, et al. Comparison of NIV-NAVA and NCPAP in facilitating extubation for very preterm infants. BMC Pediatr 2019;19(1):298.

60. De Luca D, Carnielli VP, Conti G, et al. Noninvasive high-frequency oscillatory ventilation through nasal prongs: bench evaluation of efficacy and mechanics. Intensive Care Med 2010;36(12):2094–100.

61. Centorrino R, Dell'Orto V, Gitto E, et al. Mechanics of nasal mask-delivered HFOV in neonates: a physiologic study. Pediatr Pulmonol 2019;54(8):1304–10.

62. Dumas De La Roque E, Bertrand C, Tandonnet O, et al. Nasal high-frequency percussive ventilation versus nasal continuous positive airway pressure in transient tachypnea of the newborn: a pilot randomized controlled trial (NCT00556738). Pediatr Pulmonol 2011;46(3):218–23.

63. Li J, Chen L, Shi Y. Nasal high-frequency oscillatory ventilation versus nasal continuous positive airway pressure as primary respiratory support strategies for respiratory distress syndrome in preterm infants: a systematic review and meta-analysis. Eur J Pediatr 2022;181(1):215–23.

64. Wang K, Zhou X, Gao S, et al. Noninvasive high-frequency oscillatory ventilation versus nasal intermittent positive pressure ventilation for preterm infants as an extubation support: a systematic review and meta-analysis. Pediatr Pulmonol. Mar 2023;58(3):704–11.

65. Keel J, De Beritto T, Ramanathan R, et al. Nasal high-frequency jet ventilation (NHFJV) as a novel means of respiratory support in extremely low birth weight infants. J Perinatol 2021;41(7):1697–703.

66. Taha DK, Kornhauser M, Greenspan JS, et al. High flow nasal cannula use is associated with increased morbidity and length of hospitalization in extremely low birth weight infants. J Pediatr 2016;173:50–5.e1.

67. Roberts CT, Owen LS, Manley BJ, et al. Nasal high-flow therapy for primary respiratory support in preterm infants. N Engl J Med 2016;375(12):1142–51.

68. Murki S, Singh J, Khant C, et al. High-flow nasal cannula versus nasal continuous positive airway pressure for primary respiratory support in preterm infants with respiratory distress: a randomized controlled trial. Neonatology 2018;113(3): 235–41.

69. Hodgson KA, Wilkinson D, De Paoli AG, et al. Nasal high flow therapy for primary respiratory support in preterm infants. Cochrane Database Syst Rev 2023;5(5): CD006405.

70. Manley BJ, Arnolda GRB, Wright IMR, et al. Nasal high-flow therapy for newborn infants in special care nurseries. N Engl J Med 2019;380(21):2031–40.

71. Uchiyama A, Okazaki K, Kondo M, et al. Randomized controlled trial of high-flow nasal cannula in preterm infants after extubation. Pediatrics 2020;146(6).

Monitoring SpO$_2$
The Basics of Retinopathy of Prematurity (Back to Basics) and Targeting Oxygen Saturation

Augusto Sola, MD[a,*], Leslie Altimier, DNP, RN, NE-BC, MSN, BSN[b],
María Teresa Montes Bueno, RN[c], Cristian Emanuel Muñoz, RN[d]

KEYWORDS

- ROP • SpO$_2$ • Hypoxemia • Hyperoxemia • Oxidative stress • Preterm newborn
- Intention to treat

KEY POINTS

- Normal noninvasive pulse oximetry (SpO$_2$) in room air (fractional inspired oxygen [Fio$_2$] 21%) is 95% to 100%.
- Tissue oxygenation is complex and depends on many factors other than SpO$_2$, including hemoglobin concentration and quality, cardiac output, peripheral vascular resistance, systemic blood flow, O$_2$ delivery, microcirculation, and others.
- SpO$_2$ greater than 95% to 96% when breathing supplemental O$_2$ can be associated with hyperoxemia.
- Antioxidant capacity is decreased in newborns, more so in preterm infants.
- Excess oxygen is a neonatal health hazard and hyperoxemia should be prevented from the delivery room and throughout all the hospital stay.
- The fluctuation between hypoxemia and hyperoxemia and reperfusion events is extremely noxious.

INTRODUCTION

This review focuses on the most current methods, evidence, and controversies in clinical practice regarding the basics of retinopathy of prematurity (ROP) and pulse oximetry (SpO$_2$) monitoring in neonates.

The content in this review is divided into different topics, as follows:.

- Brief historical aspects of oxygen discovery and first infants reported with ROP
- Basic and up-to-date characteristics of ROP

[a] Iberoamerican Society of Neonatology (SIBEN), 2244 Newbury Drive, Wellington, FL 3341, USA; [b] Cardinal Glennon Children's Hospital, 1465 South Grand Avenue, St. Louis, MO 63104, USA; [c] Iberoamerican Society of Neonatology (SIBEN), Calle Villa de Marín n 37-1D, Madrid 28029, Spain; [d] Iberoamerican Society of Neonatology (SIBEN), Belgrano 378 -D8, San Luis, Argentina
* Corresponding author.
E-mail address: augusto.Sola@siben.net

Crit Care Nurs Clin N Am 36 (2024) 69–98
https://doi.org/10.1016/j.cnc.2023.08.004
0899-5885/24/© 2023 Elsevier Inc. All rights reserved.
ccnursing.theclinics.com

- ○ Risk factors, epidemics
- ○ Localization (zones I–III of the eye), extension (in "clock hours"), and severity stages [1–5] of ROP
- ○ Primary prevention of ROP—Nursing role
- ○ Ophthalmologic screening—Nursing role
- ○ Treatment of ROP
- ○ SpO$_2$ monitoring
- ○ Intention to treat and target ranges for SpO$_2$ in the delivery room and newborn intensive care unit (NICU). Pitfalls of cyanosis for the diagnosis of hypoxemia or normoxemia.
- Some concepts of the physiology of tissue oxygenation
- Oxygen damage

As O$_2$ is a very potent drug often used inappropriately in the clinical environment, its administration needs to be improved in neonatal care. Therefore, the authors will emphasize on clinical concepts and practice implications with the main objective of decreasing morbidities associated with excess O$_2$ use.

BRIEF HISTORICAL ASPECTS OF OXYGEN DISCOVERY AND FIRST INFANTS REPORTED WITH RETINOPATHY OF PREMATURITY (ROP)

Oxygen (O$_2$) was discovered for the first time by a Swedish chemist, Carl Wilhelm Scheele, in 1772. Joseph Priestly, an English chemist, independently discovered oxygen in 1774 and published his findings the same year, 3 years before Scheele published. Antoine Lavoisier, a French chemist, also discovered oxygen in 1775, and was the first to recognize it as an element and coined its name "oxygen", which comes from a Greek word that means "acid-former." However, it is Priestley who is credited with the discovery of oxygen. [1,2]

Since the mid- 1940s, the history of O$_2$ use in newborn infants has been pretty intricate and inundated with misconceptions and errors and continues to be so in 2023. Wilson and colleagues showed that periodic breathing was almost completely eliminated using fractional inspired oxygen (FiO$_2$)$_2$ of 70%. [3] The authors cautioned against moving to the use of oxygen without controls and restrictions, but the American Academy of Pediatrics and other researchers liberally promoted its use. And so, … what happened … unfortunately happened. Theodore L. Terry, in 1942, described the first cases of ROP in extremely premature infants in Boston. At that time, he described a "grayish white opaque membrane behind each crystalline lens." The term "retrolental fibroplasia" was devised in 1941 by Dr. Harry H. Messenger of Boston, for use by Dr Terry. [4–9]

BASICS AND UP-TO-DATE CHARACTERISTICS OF ROP

Retinopathy of prematurity (ROP) is one of the leading, yet largely preventable cause of childhood blindness in the United States and worldwide. [10–13] Globally, at least 50,000 children are blind every year as a result of ROP and in the United States, even with many advances in ROP treatment, approximately 600 premature infants become legally blind each year. [10–13]

ROP is a vasoproliferative disorder of the immature retina that occurs most frequently in preterm infants. ROP can develop when the immature retinal blood vessels have not reached the edge of the retina, known as the ora serrata. It is multifactorial, [12,13] and several risk factors have been described. [14–18] They are summarized in **Box 1.**

> **Box 1**
> **Risk factors associated with the development of ROP**
>
> Main factors: prematurity, low birth weight, excessive O$_2$ administration, and poor weight gain and quality of neonatal hospital care received during early postnatal life.
>
> Other:
> - Impaired growth and low weight gain
> - Chorioamnionitis and sepsis (bacterial and *Candida*)
> - Mechanical ventilation
> - Respiratory distress
> - Blood transfusions
> - Anemia
> - Surfactant
> - Use of late postnatal steroids (2.9-fold increased odds ratio for severe ROP)

In **Fig. 1**, the authors show a schematic representation of the normal vasculature of the normal retina (to the right of the figure) and the vasoproliferative aberration in ROP (to the left)

ROP represents the leading cause of childhood blindness and it has been described worldwide in 3 "epidemics" [12] (**Fig. 2**).

ROP was classified according to the International Committee for the Classification of ROP (ICROP) in 1984 and revised in 2005 with a review in 2017. [19–23] ICROP described the disease according to its location, extension, and severity. For the

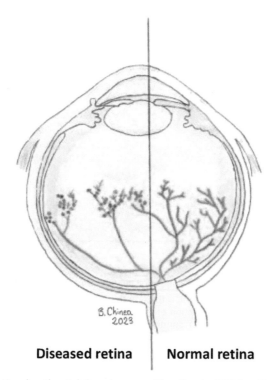

Diseased retina | **Normal retina**

Fig. 1. Normal retina (on the right) and vasoproliferation in ROP (on the left).

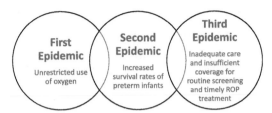

Fig. 2. The 3 "epidemics" of ROP.

location, the retina is divided into 3 zones (**Table 1**). The extent of disease is recorded as the total clock hours involved, not just the contiguous sectors (**Fig. 3**).

The severity is classified into 5 stages, and also in "plus disease," threshold ROP, and aggressive posterior retinopathy of prematurity (APROP) (**Table 2**).

The 5 stages of ROP are shown in **Fig. 4** in a schematic form.

As mentioned earlier, in **Table 1** and **Fig. 3**, the extension of ROP is based on "clock hours," and localization is divided according to the zone of the eye. In general, ROP in zone I (central zone) is more likely to progress and become more severe than ROP in zones II or III. In addition to the 5 stages of severity of ROP, 1 to 5, "plus disease, "threshold ROP, and APROP can be present, as described in **Table 2. Fig. 5** shows in a schematic way what would be considered stage 3 of ROP severity affecting zone II, threshold ROP, and "plus disease." The extension of ROP affects many clock hours, which the scheme shows in the light-shaded areas. In the left eye, the extension is 5 contiguous clock hours (from 6 to 11 hours), and in the right eye, there is a total of 8 clock hours involved (not just contiguous sectors).

PRIMARY PREVENTION OF ROP

Nurses are the main caregivers in NICUs and play a vital role in the prevention and management of ROP. [23] Obviously, a multidisciplinary team approach that includes obstetricians, neonatologists, ophthalmologists, pediatricians, respiratory therapists, other disciplines, and parents is necessary.

ROP is considered an indicator of the quality of neonatal hospital care, especially nursing care. Standard neonatal care practices, coupled with adequate education, infrastructure, and availability of resources like SpO_2 monitors, O_2 blenders, and continuous positive airway pressure systems, can influence ROP prevention and outcomes.

Nursing care practices for primary prevention of ROP include what has been called "POINTS": P-pain control, O-judicious use of oxygen, I-infection control measures,

Table 1
Localization and extension of ROP
Localization: Three Concentric Zones (I, II, III) Centered on the Papilla (see Fig. 3)

Zone I: is central, a small circle of retina around the optic disc. The radius of the circle is twice the distance from the macula to the center of the optic disc	Zone II: is the ring-shaped section of the retina surrounding zone I, which extends to the ora serrata on the nasal side	Zone III: is the remaining crescent-shaped zone located on the temporal side outside of zone II

Extension - Recorded as clock hours, in twelve 30° or 1-h sections (see **Fig. 3**)

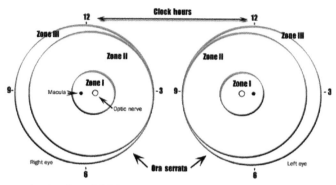

Fig. 3. Zones and extension of ROP.

N-adequate nutrition, T-thermoregulation, and S-supportive care. In **Box 2** the authors summarize several of these points.

OPHTHALMOLOGIC SCREENING

The implementation of screening programs is essential in order to diagnose cases of ROP that can be treated so that opportunities are not missed and long-term outcomes are improved. [23-28]

Table 2				
Severity of ROP: Stages, "plus disease," threshold ROP and APROP				
Stage 1	**Stage 2**	**Stage 3**	**Stage 4**	**Stage 5**
A thin and white demarcation line that separates the vascular from the avascular retina.	A visible ridge or crest, a white/pink cord that stands out on the retina	Blood vessels in the ridge. Extraretinal fibrovascular proliferation, with neo vessels and fibrous tissue into the vitreous cavity. It can be mild, moderate or severe.	Sub-total or partial retinal detachment. 4a: extrafoveal, does not affect the fovea (macula) 4b: foveal: detached macula	Total retinal detachment
"Plus + disease"	Dilation and tortuosity of the posterior pole vessels in 2 quadrants. It can accompany any of the stages above. Existence of an arteriovenous shunt. It indicates greater severity and poor prognosis.			
Threshold ROP	A condition with 50% risk of retinal detachment if left untreated. It includes ROP in zone 1 or zone 2 with more than 5 contiguous or 8 cumulative clock hours of stage 3 ROP			
Aggressive posterior retinopathy of prematurity (APROP)	A distinct variant of ROP; a severe but rare form characterized by fast progression to an advanced stage with flat neovascularization in zone 1 or zone 2. It is characterized by severe plus disease, flat neovascularization in zone 1 or posterior zone 2, intraretinal shunting, hemorrhages, and a rapid progression to retinal detachment. It does not respect various stages and can rapidly lead to blindness if untreated.			

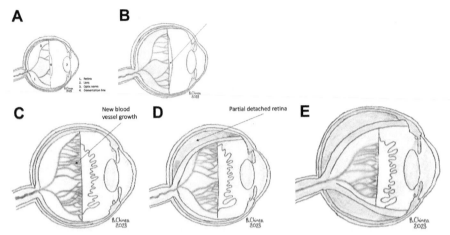

Fig. 4. (*A*) Stage 1 ROP. (*B*) Stage 2 ROP. The arrow shows a thicker and wider demarcation line that forms a ridge. (*C*) Stage 3 ROP with new blood vessel formation. (*D*) Stage 4 ROP with a partial detachment of the retina. (*E*) ROP Stage 5: Complete retinal detachment.

Screening must be done with indirect binocular ophthalmoscopy and performed by an experienced ophthalmologist who knows exactly all of the challenges of such a retinal examination. Screening programs are not easy to implement and must take into consideration the gestational age at birth to adequately schedule the timing of ophthalmologic examinations and to ensure there are no missed opportunities for treatment. **Table 3** summarizes some of the key points to consider when implementing ROP screening programs.

Fortunately, most infants do not have severe stages of ROP, and about 80% resolve spontaneously, with regression of the disease. Only the remaining 20% present some

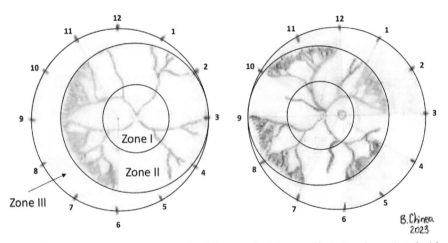

Fig. 5. Threshold ROP in zone II, stage 3, with many clock hours affected and associated with "plus disease."

Box 2
Summary of important aspects involved in primary prevention of ROP

Pain and stress control
  Management of O$_2$
  Alarms always operative
  Prevention and rapid treatment of apneic episodes
  Avoid hypoxia–hyperoxia reperfusion
  Adequate nutrition and breast milk.
  Thermoregulation
  Neurodevelopment
  Minimal interventions
  Optimal sleep cycles
  Minimal blood draws to prevent anemia and transfusions
  Infection prevention

---

degree of scar disease, passing from a phase of vascular proliferation to a fibrotic phase.

NURSING ROLE IN ROP SCREENING

Nursing staff must actively participate before, during, and after the ophthalmologic examination, [23] according to the points described in **Table 4**

It is important to know the expected time for the ophthalmologic examination in order to administer ophthalmic medication that produces mydriasis early enough so that an adequate funduscopic examination can be performed according to the protocol (see **Table 5**).

TREATMENT OF ROP. LASER AND ANTI-VASCULAR ENDOTHELIAL GROWTH FACTOR (VEGF)

Many babies with ROP have mild cases and get better without treatment. However, some babies have advanced ROP and need laser photocoagulation or ablation of the avascular retina to keep ROP from getting worse. Many studies have addressed therapeutic options. [29–36] Laser photocoagulation is the gold standard for treatment of ROP. [30–33] The milder forms of ROP have a regression rate of up to 94.11% with laser, while more severe forms, including APROP may show good regression with laser in only about 54.2% of eyes.

All eyes with plus disease and threshold disease are to be treated. Randomized clinical trials in infants with high-risk prethreshold ROP showed that earlier treatment using peripheral ablation of the avascular retina had significantly reduced unfavorable outcomes to a clinically important degree, with improved visual acuity and retinal structure compared with conventional treatment. Therefore, it is important to provide early treatment to protect vision.

Infants less than 500 g at birth are at high risk for developing prethreshold ROP and later for developing strabismus, nystagmus, high myopia, and abnormal retinal structure. These infants should, therefore, receive continued long-term follow-up. [22]

There are 2 types of retinal surgery for babies with partially or completely detached retinas (stages 4 or 5). One is scleral buckle surgery, where a band supports the detached retina until the eye starts growing normally, then the band is removed.

The other type of surgery is a vitrectomy, where small openings in the eye wall are made to remove most of the vitreous fluid, which is replaced with saline solution, and

Table 3
Key points to consider in ROP screening programs

Program Entry Criteria	First Evaluation
• All Newborns < 1500 g or < 31 wk gestational age (GA)[a]	Newborns < 27 wk at birth: at 31 wk post-conceptional age Newborns > 27 wk at birth: at 4 wk of age
• Newborns 31–33 wk GA requiring mechanical ventilation or elevated or prolonged Fio$_2$ (>7 d)	Within 1–3 wk of postnatal age
• Newborns > 33 wk GA who have received O$_2$ or present aggravating factors	Between the first and second postnatal week to confirm if the vascularization of the retina has been completed normally

Follow-up examinations
• Weekly or even more frequently if:
  ○ Stage 3 ROP in any retinal zone
  ○ Any stage of ROP in posterior Zone I or Zone II
  ○ Presence of plus disease
  ○ Presence or suspicion of posterior aggressive ROP
  ○ Immature vascularization in posterior Zone I or Zone II
• Every 1 to 2 weeks:
  ○ Immature vascularization in posterior Zone II
  ○ Stage 2 ROP in Zone II
  ○ Uncertainty if ROP in Zone I has regressed
• Every 2 weeks:
  ○ Stage 1 of ROP in Zone II
  ○ Immature vascularization in Zone II
• Every 3 weeks
  ○ Stage 1 or 2 in Zone III
  ○ Regression of ROP in Zone III

Examinations have to continue until the retina is fully vascularized, or at least to 34–36 wk post-conceptional age, depending on the infant. It has been shown that in infants < 500 g, median postmenstrual age for diagnosis of all prethreshold ROP was 36.1 wk GA, but earlier (35.1 wk GA) for eyes that developed high-risk prethreshold ROP. Thus, eye examinations should continue until at least that time. [22]

[a] In a 2020, 2 large cohort studies suggested somewhat different recommendations for evidence-based screening criteria for type 1 ROP. [28] They included all infants with gestational age less than 28 wk or birth weight less than 1051 g (g) and all larger preterm infants with poor weight gain defined as: weight gain less than 120 g during age 10 to 19 d, weight gain less than 180 g during age 20 to 29 d, or weight gain less than 170 g during age 30 to 39 d; or hydrocephalus. In the combined G-ROP-1 and G-ROP-2 cohort of 11,463 infants, the G-ROP criteria predicted 677 of 677 cases of type 1 ROP (sensitivity, 100%; 95% CI, 99.4%–100%), reducing the number of infants receiving examinations by 32.5% (n = 3730). This provides evidence-based screening criteria that have higher sensitivity and higher specificity (fewer infants receiving examinations) for stage 1 ROP than currently recommended guidelines. [28]

the scar tissue on the retina is removed. Laser treatment may also be performed to treat the retina and seal it into position. The goal of ROP surgery is to keep ROP from getting worse and to prevent blindness. Even with surgery, some babies with ROP will still have severe vision loss or blindness.

Anti-vascular endothelial growth factor (VEGF) drugs, like bevacizumab, ranibizumab and others, injected into the baby's eye have also been used for ROP treatment. [34–36] If edema is located in the center of the macula, these injections may be superior to laser. However, supplemental laser treatment may be necessary to seal leaks after the injections begin to take effect. If macular edema is not located in the center of the retina, the laser alone may protect against loss of vision. Even in cases of APROP, laser should still

Table 4 Nursing roles in screening for ROP	
Before ROP screening	• Know the Institutional screening program. • Record birth weight and GA. • Monitor weight gain. • Detect and select babies that require screening. • Advise parents on the procedure. • Place the baby in a calm and comfortable position. • Perform pupil dilation for the examination. (**Table 5** of Medication)
During	• Good hand washing of all team members. • Have the material for screening ready. (see **Table 5** of materials) • Position the baby in a swaddled and comfortable position. • Assess, identify, and manage pain. Use non-pharmacological measures. (**Box 3**) • Use anesthetic drops prior to the ophthalmologic examination. (see **Table 5**) • Record infant's tolerance during the procedure and if any interventions were needed. • Monitor vital signs: blood pressure, heart rate, and SpO$_2$.
After	• Strictly control and monitor newborns, since they tend to be uncomfortable and may have less tolerance for feedings. • Place the baby in a calm and comfortable position. • Protect the newborn from ambient light and excessive stimulation. • Record the baby's tolerance to the procedure. • Carry out the required documentation. • Set a date and time for the next screening examination.

be considered as a primary modality of treatment as it has been shown to have an overall success rate of 94%, [34] it is a one-time treatment without the concern of systemic side effects and recurrent/persistent avascular zones of anti-VEGF drugs. Other studies have shown that the evidence for anti-VEGF treatment is of low or very low quality due to the risk of detection bias and other biases. [35,36] For example, intravitreal bevacizumab/ranibizumab, when used as monotherapy, reduces the risk of refractive errors during childhood but does not reduce the risk of retinal detachment or recurrence of ROP in infants with type 1 ROP. The effects on other critical outcomes and, more importantly, the long-term systemic adverse effects of the drugs are not known. [35] VEGF inhibitors seem to be associated with low recurrence rates and ocular complication rates. They may have the benefit of potentially allowing the preservation of the visual field, as well as lower rates of myopia. However, concerns remain, especially about possible

Table 5 Medications and material for ophthalmologic screening	
Medication for Ophthalmologic Examination	**Material**
Start 1 h before the examination. Phenylephrine ophthalmic solution (100 mg/mL eye drops) diluted to $\frac{1}{4}$ (2.5%): 1 drop in each eye Cycloplegic (cyclopentolate eye drops 10 mg/mL) diluted to ½ (0.5%): 1 drop in each eye. Repeat after 10–15 min. Local anesthetic: Proparacaine hydrochloride 0.5%. The anesthetic action begins 20 s after the drop is applied.	Indirect binocular ophthalmoscope Sterile material: • Blepharostats for preterm infants • Scleral indenters

> **Box 3**
> **Non-pharmacological pain management, sedation, and analgesia for ROP screening**
>
> - Administration of oral saccharose (sucrose) 24% and/or breast milk—2 minutes before starting the procedure.
> - Containment measures and non-nutritive sucking with a pacifier during the procedure.
> - Reduce light and auditory stress.
> - Monitor vital signs and signs of pain or discomfort.
> - Evaluate repeated doses of saccharose or breast milk according to assessment.
> - Assessment and prescription by the neonatologist of necessary systemic pharmacologic analgesia (ie,: morphine, fentanyl)

systemic complications. [36] In summary, anti-VEGF injections are not as effective as laser surgery and have potential adverse effects.

SpO_2 MONITORING IN NEONATES AND INTENTION TO TREAT

SpO_2 monitors were entered into practice in the 1980s with the main goal of promptly detecting hypoxemia. A few years later they were considered the "fifth vital sign." However, the routine implementation of SpO_2 monitors occurred without randomized trials and, more importantly, without education of neonatal bedside care providers about some known physiologic principles, such as the changing relation between O_2 and hemoglobin (Hb), arterial Po_2 (Pao_2), O_2 saturation, and the oxyhemoglobin dissociation curve. [37]

HOW DO SATURATION MONITORS FUNCTION?

In 1972, Takuo Aoyagi, an electrical engineer at Nihon Kohden company in Tokyo, realized that pulsatile changes could be used to compute saturation from the ratio of ratios of pulse changes in the red and infrared wavelengths. [38] His ideas, equations, and instruments were adapted, improved, and successfully marketed by Minolta in 1978, to monitor SpO_2 non-invasively and without the need for calibration. This stimulated other firms to further improve and market pulse oximeters worldwide in the mid-1980s. [38] Since then, many changes have occurred.

Oxygenated hemoglobin (Hbo_2) and deoxygenated or reduced Hb absorb and transmit discrete wavelengths of light, for the red light around 660 nm and for the infrared light around 940 nm. This is according to a physical property unique to each molecular species called the extinction coefficient. The physics of pulse oximetry has been based on the Beer–Lambert law, which takes into consideration the extinction coefficient, the concentration, and the optical path length.

The SpO_2 sensor or probe consists of 2 light-emitting diodes (LED), 1 for red light and 1 for infrared, and of a photodiode detector. For best performance, the LEDs and the detector must be placed on opposite sides of a translucent perfused site. In neonates, the hand or foot is commonly used. The photodiode measures 3 different light levels: red light, infrared light, and may also be affected by the ambient light level. To avoid decubitus injuries due to the prolonged use of sensors, it is recommended to change the site every 6-8-12 hours. In newborns, during the transition and when right to left shunt is suspected, the sensor should be preductal (right hand, **Fig. 6**A). In all other cases, the feet can be used (**Fig. 6**B), as well as the left hand.

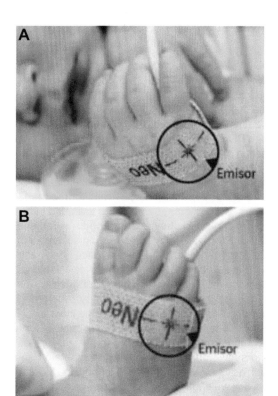

Fig. 6. Preductal (*A*) and Postductal (*B*) position of sensor.

SpO$_2$ records only the transmitted light values of the added volume of arterial blood that surges through the tissues with each arterial pulse. This is called the pulsating arterial component [AC]. The light absorbed changes as the amount of blood in the tissue bed changes and as the relative amounts of Hbo$_2$ and Hb change. In addition, there is the non-moving static component [DC]. This includes tissue, bone, blood vessels, fluids, and skin, as well as the LED intensity, the detector response, and the relatively low-frequency venous blood. By dividing AC by DC for each LED, the transmission of light is normalized and calibration would not be required. Thus, through spectrophotometric methods, SpO$_2$ monitors measure Hbo$_2$ and Hb by absorption of red and infrared light.

The relative proportions of Hbo$_2$ and Hb are detected by SpO$_2$ monitors according to the normalized ratio of light transmitted between the red and infrared lights, or the R/Ir ratio. Essentially, this means that at the photodetector, the ratio of R/Ir for both AC and DC correlates with SpO$_2$. This needs a "look-up table" to compute the existing R/Ir ratio to SpO$_2$. For example, when the R/Ir ratio is 2.50, the SpO$_2$ is 0%; when R/Ir ratio is 1.50, the SpO2 is 40%; and when the R/Ir ratio reaches 0.40, the SpO$_2$ is 100%.

Based on the original work of Aoyagi, it was assumed, though incorrectly, that only arterial blood pulsates (or moves) within the measuring site. An important breakthrough was when Joe Kiani and Mohamed Diab invented pulse oximetry with signal extraction technology (SET) in 1995, with the ability to separate the arterial signal from noise. This allowed for increased accuracy and much more precision in SpO$_2$ measurements when there is motion and/or low perfusion, decreasing or completely eliminating sources of noise that affect SpO$_2$ readings. [39]

SPECIFICITY, SENSITIVITY, BIAS, AND FALSE ALARMS OF DIFFERENT SpO$_2$ MONITORS

SpO$_2$ monitors available in the market have differences in their performance, specificity, and sensitivity and there are many publications in relation to this topic. [39–49] For example, Baquero, and colleagues [45] described significant improvements in SpO$_2$ readings in the delivery room during acute resuscitation when signal extraction technology (SET) was used compared to other monitors, and Castillo and colleagues [46] showed that severe ROP was reduced between 54% and 58% in 2 different centers with the implementation of Masimo SET (Masimo, Irvine, CA) as compared to Nellcor SpO$_2$ (Medtronic, Irvine CA) monitors. Robertson and Hoffman [47] showed several years ago that with low signal quality or during hypoxemia, the new devices are not clinically equivalent to each other. Masimo SET monitor reported less data questionable than Nellcor in this study. Accuracy was also validated in animal models of low perfusion. [48] A few years ago, the authors performed a comprehensive state-of-the-art review that described in detail many factors of significance in pulse oximetry. [49]

Precision is a standard deviation of the difference. Accuracy is the root mean squared error (A$_{RMS}$*). A$_{RMS}$ accuracy is a statistical calculation of the difference between device measurements and reference measurements. The Signal Extraction Technology – SET sensors have the best accuracy reported (1.5% A$_{RMS}$) to the FDA. There are also significant differences in the sensors available in the market, but their description exceeds the scope of this manuscript. The major differences between monitors are summarized in **Box 4**.

Most SpO$_2$ monitors have only 2 wavelengths and therefore they cannot measure dyshemoglobins such as COHb and MetHb. Differently, the Masimo rainbow SET platform, which employs 8 wavelengths, has the unique ability to measure the level of carbon monoxide in the blood, dyshemoglobins (carboxyhemoglobin, methemoglobin), and total hemoglobin concentration. [50,51]

Finally, different monitors also have different specifications in averaging time, alarm delay, and response sensitivity. [52] With Masimo SET, an average time between 2 and 6 seconds is recommended depending on whether the monitor is being used during a resuscitation (shorter average time) or in the NICU.

Many factors can affect the R/Ir sensed by the photodetector and therefore can interfere with the accuracy of SpO$_2$ monitors, regardless of which monitor is being used (**Table 6**).

In addition to all that is aforementioned, the recommendation made by many manufacturers to improve reliability is to first have the SpO$_2$ monitor turned on with its cable in place (but not connected to the patient's sensor cable), second to place the sensor on the child's right hand, and third, finally connect it to the cable. If the SpO$_2$ monitor cable is plugged into the patient's sensor cable before being placed on the infant, it will be searching for and reading an SpO$_2$ reading from the ambient environment, which can be misleading to staff. In summary, ensure the sensor and cable are connected last to minimize the time the sensor is trying to pick up signals from the environment (and not the application site).

NORMAL AND ABNORMAL OXYGEN LIMITS, SpO$_2$, AND PA$_{O2}$

Normal healthy newborns breathing room air (Fio$_2$ 21%) have a Pao$_2$ of around 48 to 70 mm Hg when they are supposed to have an SpO$_2$ of 95% or above. In the past, many invasive arterial punctures were performed until continuous transcutaneous PO$_2$ (Tc Po$_2$) measurements became available. This was markedly transformed when non-invasive SpO$_2$ monitors that do not require calibration became available.

Box 4
Differences in SpO$_2$ monitors
Number of wave lengths.
Sensitivity.
Specificity.
Bias.
Percent of false alarms.
Signal extraction Technology – SET

However, most care providers understand better arterial partial pressure of oxygen (Pao)$_2$ values than SpO$_2$ values. Unfortunately, many bedside health care providers assumed that the normal SpO$_2$ values (at 95% or above) described in newborns' breathing room air (Fio$_2$ 21%) were to be maintained in sick newborns treated with supplemental O$_2$. This was absolutely mistaken, as SpO$_2$ monitors were designed to detect hypoxemia but not to detect hyperoxemia.

INTENTION TO TREAT OR "TARGET" SpO$_2$

The intention to treat ("target SpO$_2$") in infants breathing supplemental O$_2$ should not include SpO$_2$ values associated with potential hyperoxia or possible hypoxia and also must aim to avoid recurring periods of hypoxemia–hyperoxemia reperfusion, starting from the time of birth.

SpO$_2$ IN THE DELIVERY ROOM

During the transitional period, the O$_2$ saturation increases slowly over 10 to 15 minutes. Normal SpO$_2$ is less than 70% initially. Many uncompromised neonates breathing room air do not reach preductal O$_2$ saturation greater than 90% until approximately 10 minutes after birth, or even later. This happens a little bit sooner in term infants than in preterm newborns. It is not fully known what a normal SpO$_2$ is in very preterm

Table 6	
Factors that may interfere with the accuracy of SpO$_2$ monitors	
Noise, motion artifacts and excessive patient movement[a]	Ambient light
	Dark-skinned populations[b]
Low perfusion or pulse pressure (shock, vasoconstriction, hypotension)[a]	Low peripheral temperature
	Signal quality
Sensor mispositioning	Phototherapy in some monitors
Venous oxygen saturation	Severe anemia
Cold extremities—Hypothermia	Less accuracy when saturation is < 70%–75%

[a] As mentioned earlier, Masimo SET technology allows more accurate readings in cases of low peripheral perfusion, hypothermia, hypotension, low cardiac output, vasoconstrictor drugs, movement, and situations in which there is an increased venous pulse wave that is,: some drugs and right heart failure.
[b] A recent study found that Masimo SET Pulse Oximetry has no difference in accuracy or bias between black people and white people.[53]

infants during their transition to extrauterine life and whether the SpO_2 values are different for those who require resuscitation.

Several authors have addressed the progressively increasing SpO_2 values in newborn infants breathing room air according to the age in minutes after birth, and the use of O_2 in the delivery room and among them.[54–66]: The authors summarize the findings in (**Table 7**).

As seen, the preductal SpO_2 of 95% to 100% is not reached for several minutes.

Based on this information, the SpO_2 target in the delivery room for infants receiving supplemental O_2 should not be the same as it is in the NICU, which will be discussed later.

USE OF O_2 IN THE DELIVERY ROOM

An exact supply of O_2 is necessary to avoid the negative consequences of hypoxia or hyperoxia in the delivery room. What Fio_2 to use for the first steps of neonatal resuscitation is a question that has been answered pretty accurately for term infants, but not as precisely for preterm infants.[67–72] The use of room air (21% O_2) instead of high concentrations of inhaled O_2 has been shown to be safe and effective with a decreased risk of neonatal mortality for term and late preterm infants. The current recommendations of the American Heart Association are to use of 21% O_2 for the initial resuscitation of newborns greater than 35 weeks of gestation. For preterm newborns less than 34 to 35 weeks and, more so, for those less than 30 to 32 weeks gestation, it is still "an unanswered riddle" whether the most accurate Fio_2 to use in the initial steps of resuscitation is 21%, 30%, or 40%. [72]

When resuscitation is required, preductal SpO_2 (right hand) monitoring should be started as soon as possible with the intention to treat maintaining the SpO_2 ranges mentioned earlier (see **Table 7**, **Fig. 7**), to avoid not only hypoxemia but also hyperoxemia. Therefore, it is always recommended to monitor SpO_2 when there is suspicion of hypoxemia, and also when the administration of supplemental O_2 is initiated, and/or when resuscitation is required and the administration of positive-pressure ventilation lasts for more than a few breaths.

Hyperoxemia in the delivery room, even for a few minutes, is dangerous and has been associated with pediatric cancer, ROP, and other morbidities, as the authors describe in this review.

CYANOSIS

Skin or tongue color is not reliable for detecting hypoxemia.[73–75] Cyanosis is the bluish discoloration of skin and mucosae. Many times, clinicians make the diagnosis of cyanosis, but there is no hypoxemia. More frequently even, there could be abnormally low SpO_2 and no visible cyanosis. Several factors are responsible for this and are summarized in **Box 5**.

Table 7		
Summary of progressively increasing SpO_2 during the transition to extrauterine life		
Post-natal Age	SpO_2 in Term Infants	SpO_2 in Preterm Infants
3 min	55%–80%	55%–75%
5 min	75%–90%	75%–85%
10 min	90%–97%	85%–90%

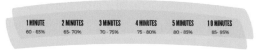

1 MINUTE	2 MINUTES	3 MINUTES	4 MINUTES	5 MINUTES	10 MINUTES
60 - 65%	65- 70%	70 - 75%	75 - 80%	80 - 85%	85- 95%

Fig. 7. Target preductal SpO$_2$ in the delivery room for term and preterm infants breathing supplemental O$_2$ (based on many publications).

For cyanosis to occur, there has to be a concentration of reduced or desaturated Hb of at least greater than or equal to 3 g/dL. **Fig. 8** shows 2 infants with different concentrations of total Hb. The one on the top of the figure has a concentration of total Hb of 17.5 g/dL. This infant will have greater or equal to 3 g/dL of desaturated Hb when SpO$_2$ is 83% or less (i.e. 17% of desaturated Hb). No clinician would be able to detect real and true cyanosis before that happens.

On the other infant with a total Hb of 13.5 g/dL, the desaturation has to be at least 22% for the concentration of reduced Hb to be at least 3 g/dL. Therefore, cyanosis will be visible only when SpO$_2$ is less than 78%. The ineffectiveness of the human eye to clinically detect desaturation less than 95% is considered a "blind spot" **Fig. 8**.

In the example (see **Fig. 8**), for desaturated Hb to be greater than 3 g/dL, the SpO$_2$ has to be as low as 83% in one of the infants and 78% or less in the other one. Clearly, the ability to detect cyanosis is worse at lower hemoglobin values. It is essential to keep this in mind to avoid significant and/or persistent hypoxemia, which can be easily detected with SpO$_2$ monitors.

To clarify this point further, the higher the total Hb concentration or hematocrit level, the easier it will be to see a color change. The following are 2 examples of conditions with low and high total Hb concentrations.

A baby with a total Hb concentration of 10 g/dL (or a hematocrit of approximately 30%), will need a desaturation of about 25% to 30% in order to have sufficient concentration of desaturated Hb (2,5–3.0 g/dL) for cyanosis to be perceived by all health care professionals. That is to say that, in this infant, cyanosis will clearly be visible only with an SpO$_2$ of 70% to 75%.

On the contrary, with a high total Hb concentration, cyanosis will be visible at a significantly higher SpO$_2$. For example, with a total Hb of 22 g/dL (hematocrit of approximately 66%), a sufficient concentration of desaturated Hb (2,5–3.0 g/dL) for cyanosis to occur will happen with desaturation of about 10% to 15% or SpO$_2$ of 85% to 90%

Box 5
Factors making it difficult to perceive cyanosis, even with hypoxemia

Perception of color is variable among human beings

Skin color and race

Ambient light

Infants with normal, but lower hematocrit

Anemia

"Blind spot" (see **Fig. 8**)

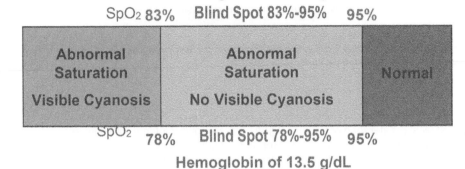

Fig. 8. Example of "blind spots" for cyanosis in the face of hypoxemia.

SpO₂ IN THE NICU

When a newborn is given supplemental O_2 in the NICU, what should the SpO_2 be when leaving the delivery room?

The authors published the first manuscript that showed that with an intention to treat aimed at avoiding SpO_2 greater than 95%, severe ROP was significantly reduced in preterm infants less than 1500 g. [76] Subsequently, a vast number of publications have addressed the topic, including review articles, prospective randomized trials, and observational studies. The authors summarize in the following paragraphs the major findings reported by some of these studies. [77–103]

Several clinical publications showed that in preterm infants breathing supplemental O_2, the objective of preventing both hypoxemia and hyperoxemia was associated with a decreased rate of severe ROP (for example, an SpO_2 between 85% and 86% for the lowest value and a high SpO_2 value of 94%). Additionally, wide-ranging arterial oxygen and SpO_2 fluctuations have been associated with ROP and the severity of ROP. [78,79]

It is of serious concern that increases in institutional SpO_2 targets in response to randomized clinical trials were associated with higher rates of severe ROP. In one study, hospitals that increased SpO_2 targets to 91% to 95% had a 3% increase in severe ROP (from 12% to 15%; aOR 5 1.25; 95% CI, 1.01–1.55; P 5 0.044) and hospitals without changes in SpO_2 targets had a 2% decrease of ROP. [92] In another recent publication, various strategies to keep infants receiving supplemental O_2 within an SpO_2 target of 91% and 95% were implemented. [94] The authors hypothesized that the incidence of severe ROP might be reduced. However, even though the SpO_2 remained within 91% to 95%, the incidence of severe ROP did not decline. [94] In another study, the higher saturation target and tighter alarm limits led to increased time with hyperoxemia, and the proportion of time with SpO_2 greater than 95% was increased by 9%. [96]

A different study compared a biphasic protocol with target SpO_2 saturations of 85% to 92% at less than 34 weeks' corrected gestational age and SpO_2 of 95% at 34 weeks gestation or older. The post-randomized trial group underwent a static 91% to 95% SpO_2 target. The biphasic oxygen standards were associated with a decreased incidence and severity of ROP without an increase in mortality. [88] Additionally, relatively high SpO_2 targeting of 91% to 95% was associated with a trend toward reduced retinal blood vessel growth. [97] Unfortunately, there is considerable variation in SpO_2

Table 8		
Acceptable and unacceptable SpO$_2$ Ranges		
Acceptable SpO$_2$ Ranges		Unacceptable SpO$_2$ Ranges
85%–93%		85%–89%
86%–94%		83%–85%
89%–94%		91%–95%
		96%–100%

targets for preterm infants in many centers; this has been well described in Italian NICUs. [98] The authors concluded that standard operating procedures and specific training for health care personnel are the main factors playing a role in the correct maintenance of recommended SpO$_2$ targets in preterm infants.

Based on the findings of the aforementioned publications and other available publications, hospitals considering using SpO$_2$ targets of 91% to 95% should anticipate no improvements or actually, an increase in the rates of severe ROP. [99]

SUMMARY

In summary, a narrow intention to treat in low ranges (i.e. SpO$_2$ target 85%–89%) should not be used clinically. Additionally, there is no evidence that a narrow SpO$_2$ target of 91% to 95% should be universally used in clinical practice for preterm infants in the initial periods of life. As mentioned earlier, this could be associated with more infants having severe ROP. Choosing wider intermediate SpO$_2$ ranges for the intention to treat allows for easier care and better compliance, and such ranges have been associated with a decreased rate of severe ROP and other potential hyperoxic damage, without an increase in morbidity or mortality.

Table 8 shows various acceptable and unacceptable SpO$_2$ ranges for intention to treat in preterm infants breathing supplemental O$_2$.

Although target SpO$_2$ values for term and preterm infants are not yet fully standardized, the concept of fluctuations rather than absolute values appears to play an increasingly important role in the occurrence of adverse events. It is almost impossible to keep preterm newborns breathing supplemental O$_2$ within the desired intention-to-treat at all times, and the percent of time outside the desired intention-to-treat is much higher when narrower ranges are used, causing more episodes of hypoxia–hyperoxia reperfusion with potential serious negative consequences. Implementing wider target ranges for SpO$_2$ may be more practically and lead to better results; however, more studies are needed to determine the impact on mortality and neurologic disability.

Currently, some monitors offer the possibility of seeing how the SpO$_2$ has evolved by observing histograms of SpO$_2$ over time. In this way, quality improvement actions can be implemented to better meet the objectives of SpO$_2$ targeting, according to the clinical situation of the infant. With this method, rates of severe ROP were significantly reduced. [91]

The following photographs show histograms of actual preterm infants in the authors' NICU.

Photograph 1: SpO$_2$ 12-h histogram in a preterm baby on 0.21 Fio$_2$ and CPAP; 94% of the time SpO$_2$ is 90% to 98% (normal would be 95%–100%).

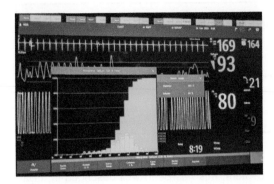

Photograph 2: SpO_2, 12-h histogram in a preterm baby on 0.25 Fio_2 and nasal ventilation; 12% of the time SpO_2 is greater than 95% (alarm had been inappropriately set at SpO_2 of 97%). Only 7% of the time the SpO_2 is less than 86%.

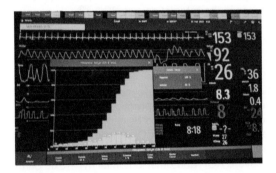

Doing everything possible to optimize SpO_2 values is not simple, but it leads to better outcomes. [92,96,101,103,104]

There are several studies that have evaluated systems of automated oxygen delivery in preterm neonates receiving supplemental O_2 with or without mechanical ventilation. [105–111] Fio_2 adjustments are made automatically and quickly, and the Fio_2 is increased or decreased mechanically according to whether the system perceives a predetermined decrease or increase in the patient's SpO_2. There are various manufacturers of this "closed loop" or automated oxygen delivery system, but all use SpO_2 monitors with SET. It has been shown that with these systems, the patient spends less percentages of time with hyperoxia and shorter periods of hypoxemia, and there is a decrease in the workload of healthcare personnel in the NICU. Closed loop or automated oxygen delivery systems are currently used widely in various European countries and other regions of the world, but no such system has been approved by the FDA for use in the United States due to concerns and potentially serious risks. Although the impact on clinical outcomes associated with automated oxygen delivery systems is yet to be proven, merely adopting the recommendations of targeting SpO_2 will not suffice. It is essential that this is achieved. Automatic titration of Fio_2 is a promising technology that helps to achieve this target; however, the clinical benefits of it are still unknown. These automatic control systems have not shown long-term benefits, and there is a concern that too many or too frequent Fio_2 changes may occur, as well as potential mechanical failures, both of which could be detrimental.

SpO$_2$ during transport: The transport of preterm newborns, either from the delivery room to the NICU, or to another hospital, represents a risk to achieving the correct oxygenation for the infant. The SpO$_2$ intention to treat during transports should be, as mentioned before in the NICU, with blended, heated, and humidified gases.

PHYSIOLOGY OF TISSUE OXYGENATION

Tissue oxygenation (TO) is essential for survival and to avoid cell death. This section summarizes the basic concepts of TO. [112–117]

Of course, TO is related to the quantity of oxygen in the atmosphere, the amount that reaches the alveoli, the diffusion through alveolar membranes, and the extent that reaches the blood.

This is summarized by the alveolar gas equation, where the arterial partial pressure of oxygen (P$_{AO_2}$) is the alveolar pressure of O$_2$, expressed in mm Hg. P$_{atm}$ is the atmospheric (or barometric) pressure, and P$_{H_2O}$ is the water vapor pressure (usually 47 mm Hg). Fio$_2$ is the fractional concentration of inspired O$_2$. In room-air, the Fio$_2$ is always 21%. At sea level, with P$_{atm}$ of about 760 mm Hg, the pressure of the inspired O$_2$ (PiO$_2$) will be about 150 mm Hg. This PiO$_2$ reaches the alveoli, where there is alveolar CO$_2$ (P$_{aco_2}$) of about 40 mm Hg. Therefore, at sea level, the P$_{AO_2}$ is about 110 mm Hg (150 mm Hg minus 40 mm Hg). The O$_2$ then diffuses into the blood. In newborn infants, the amount of intra and extrapulmonary shunting is much larger than in children and adults and this is the reason why the arterial Po$_2$ (Pao$_2$) in healthy neonates is as low as 45 or 50 mm Hg and up to 70 to 75 mm Hg, significantly lower than in adults.

In mountains and areas of the world that are many meters above sea level, the alveolar gas equation is the same, except that the P$_{atm}$ is lower, and decreases with increasing altitude. For example, at very high altitudes, the P$_{atm}$ can be 600 mm Hg. Therefore, the PiO$_2$ will only be about 125 mm Hg and the P$_{AO_2}$ 80 to 85 mm Hg. The Pao$_2$ in healthy neonates is 45 to 55 mm Hg, somewhat lower than at sea level. However, the SpO$_2$ is very similar or exactly the same. This is due to the greater binding affinity for O$_2$ of fetal hemoglobin, which is in high concentrations during neonatal life.

When a baby is breathing supplemental O$_2$, the P$_{AO_2}$ increases accordingly. If Fio$_2$ is 100%, doing the same calculations for the alveolar gas equation just mentioned, the P$_{AO_2}$ will be about 670 mm Hg, potentially poisonous for the alveolar cells. If the lungs and heart are normal, the neonatal P$_{AO_2}$ could be as high as 400 mm Hg.

Oxygenated blood returns from the lungs to the heart and is distributed throughout the body by way of systemic vasculature. O$_2$ is carried in the blood in 2 forms. The vast majority of O$_2$ in the blood is bound to hemoglobin within red blood cells, while a small amount of O$_2$ is physically dissolved in the plasma.

TO is a complex process and not easy to assess in clinical practice. [115,116] O$_2$ is released from hemoglobin in the red blood cell (RBC), diffuses across the RBC membrane into the plasma, then crosses the micro vessel wall through the interstitial fluid, eventually entering the mitochondria. Mitochondria are the primary consumers of O$_2$ and the ultimate destination of approximately 98% of the O$_2$ reaching our tissue cells. Adequate TO (normoxia) refers to the case when the tissue Po$_2$ is greater than the critical value needed for maximal mitochondrial ATP production. Inadequate TO (hypoxia) refers to the case when the Po$_2$ is below the critical value needed for mitochondrial ATP production. **Table 9** summarizes all factors involved in the process of cellular and tissue oxygenation, other than the alveolar gas equation mentioned earlier.

As it can be understood by reviewing Table 9, TO is an involved and complex process. Pao$_2$ is not really an important factor for adequate TO. Hypoxemia (low Pao$_2$)

Table 9
Factors involved in cellular and tissue oxygenation

Pao_2	Vascular Resistance
Hemoglobin (HbF Different from HbA)	Perfusion
SpO_2	O_2 Transport (DO_2)
Oxygen Content (Hb × SpO_2 + 0.003 mL)	O_2 Delivery and O_2 Consumption (Vo_2)
$Paco_2$ pH	Tissue Oxygen Diffusion Coefficient
Temperature	Various Local Phenomena: Including Local Po_2;
Glucose	Local CO_2; Local pH; Local Temperature;
Cardiac Output (minute Volume): Heart	Precapillary Sphincters; Post Capillary Venules;
Rate × Stroke or Systolic Volume	Final Distance (~10–50 μm) from Capillary to
	Mitochondria

does not necessarily cause tissue hypoxia. Additionally, tissue hypoxia can occur without hypoxemia, or even with hyperoxemia.

OXYGEN DAMAGE

Mental changes during O_2 therapy in adults with obstructive lung disease were described more than 70 years ago by Julius Comroe. [118] Since then, the potential adverse effects of providing unnecessary O_2 have expanded exponentially. [119–134] Education in oxygenation and in how oxygen is given to newborns needs to increase. Treatment with O_2 should not be considered proverbial and customary as it has been for many years since O_2 may lead to serious acute or chronic health effects (as we describe in this review). Inappropriate O_2 use is a neonatal health hazard associated with aging, DNA damage, cancer, retinopathy of prematurity, injury to the developing brain, infection, and others, as shown in **Fig. 9**. Neonatal exposure to pure O_2, even if brief, or to SpO_2 greater than 95% when breathing supplemental O_2 must be prevented as much as possible. Excess O_2 administration should be avoided at all times, including in the delivery room, the NICU, during transport, and also before, during, and after anesthesia and resuscitation.

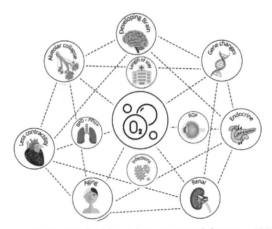

Fig. 9. Neonatal diseases associated with oxidant stress and damage. *BPD: bronchopulmonary dysplasia. PPH: persistent pulmonary hypertension.

Excessive production of free radicals (FR) and reactive oxygen species (ROS), like superoxide anions, hydroxyl radicals, hydrogen peroxide, singlet oxygen, and others, lead to progressive oxidative damage (OD), and finally cell death. OD depends on a delicate equilibrium between FR and ROS production and destruction.

There are many hazards of hyperoxemia and hyperoxia are many (see **Fig. 9**). Undesired effects of maternal, fetal, and neonatal oxidative stress involve every organ system, mitochondria, and many genes.

The body has various antioxidant systems that scavenge free radicals and ROS. They are mitochondrial, cytosolic, and peroxisomal antioxidant systems, including catalases, glutathione, and several others comprising superoxide dismutases (SODs). SODs are the primary ROS-detoxifying enzymes, but when large amounts of free O$_2$, FR, and ROS are present, the ability of these systems to prevent or repair damage is exceeded, leading to cell death or deterioration. Furthermore, antioxidant capacity is decreased in newborns, more so in preterm infants, and this exposes them to easier production of oxidant stress and damage, thus giving rise to the term "oxygen radical diseases in neonatology (ORDIN)" or oxygen radical diseases in neonatology.

The wide range of neonatal diseases associated with oxidant stress and damage are summarized in **Fig. 9** and they include intraventricular hemorrhage, periventricular leukomalacia, chronic lung disease/bronchopulmonary dysplasia, necrotizing enterocolitis, apnea of prematurity, long-term neurodevelopmental abnormalities, damage to DNA (cancer), increased infection rate, worse myocardial contractility, aging and, of course, ROP, among others.

SUMMARY AND CLINICAL PEARLS

- The history of oxygen discovery dates back to 1772 and 1974. Since then and until today, for over 250 years, the saga has been intricate, inundated with misconceptions and errors that lead to O$_2$ still being misused.
- In neonatal medicine, the first infants reported with ROP were in Boston in the 1940s. The information on the serious side effects of excess O$_2$, oxidative stress, and oxidant damage has markedly increased in the last 25 years, and several oxygen radical diseases in neonatology ("ORDIN") have been described.
- It is essential to continue to expand the knowledge and understanding of bedside care providers on O$_2$ administration and monitoring in order to avoid or minimize practices that are known to be risky. For example, fluctuations between hypoxemia and hyperoxemia and reperfusion events are extremely noxious and can be avoided.
- Most would agree that finding "the best practice" is frequently not obtainable, but eradicating a "bad practice" known to be associated with increased hazards is important and should occur. In daily clinical practice, this would be beneficial to achieving better neonatal health outcomes.
- All of us (RNs, NNPs, RTs, and MDs) must become more focused on understanding all aspects of O$_2$ administration and pulse oximetry, and on reacting properly to monitor alarms.

CLINICS CARE POINTS

- The management of O$_2$ therapy for all newborns should begin in the delivery room, in the transition period to extrauterine neonatal life, and continue in stabilization, transport, and in the NICU.

- Excess O_2 administration should be avoided at all times, including before, during, and after anesthesia and resuscitation.
- It is necessary to always use blended gases, not pure O_2 regardless of the respiratory support provided, so that the supplemental O_2 that the newborn breathes can be minimized, adjusting it to the SpO_2 intention to treat.
- In the transition period, it is advisable to monitor SpO_2 in the right hand. Subsequently, the sensor could be placed in any extremity that does not have compromised circulation.
- Quick attention to SpO_2 alarms (when they go out of range) and identifying the causes that have produced the alarm can avoid important fluctuations of SpO_2 and consequent damage by hypoxia–hyperoxia episodes.
- Change an SpO_2 monitor with false readings, false alarms, and holding periods.
- Education in oxygenation and in how oxygen is given to newborns needs to increase. O_2 may lead to serious acute or chronic health effects.
- Inappropriate O_2 use is a neonatal health hazard associated with aging, DNA damage, cancer, retinopathy of prematurity, injury to the developing brain, infection, and others.
- Normal SpO_2 when breathing room air is 95% to 100%.
- When breathing supplemental O_2, it is not acceptable to maintain SpO_2 greater than 95% to 96% and this must be prevented as much as possible.
- Neonatal exposure to pure (100%) O_2, even if brief, must be avoided.
- The intention to treat and target SpO_2 ranges in neonates breathing supplemental O_2 in the NICU, or elsewhere, should be wide. SpO_2 of 86% to 94% is usually acceptable in preterm infants.
- Low and high alarms must be set appropriately in SpO_2 monitors and should always be operative.
- One recommendation for a low SpO_2 alarm limit is about 85%.
- For infants breathing supplemental O_2, the high SpO_2 alarm depends on the intention to treat for each infant. It could be set 1% above the highest accepted SpO_2 value chosen for each infant. In preterm infants, it is usually about 94% to 95%.
- During the transition period, normal SpO_2 in room air is not 95% to 100%. It may take up to 10 minutes or more to reach those values. Therefore, the intention to treat and target SpO_2 ranges during this period should be based on accepted values according to the postnatal age in minutes.
- Cyanosis is not a reliable clinical sign for the diagnosis of hypoxemia or normoxemia, and we all have "blind spots." Screening for ROP: After each instillation of eye drops, it is recommended to maintain light pressure on the lacrimal sac for 2 minutes. This minimizes systemic absorption of drugs through the nasal mucosa that can cause hypertension, fever, tachycardia, irritability, apnea, and other side effects. This is very important in the most immature infants and in newborns with chronic lung disease.

INTERNATIONAL COMMITTEE OF MEDICAL JOURNAL EDITORS (ICMJE) AUTHORSHIP CRITERIA

A. Sola: Conception and design of the work. A. Sola, M.T. Montes Bueno, and C. Muñoz: acquisition, analysis, and interpretation of data; drafting the work and revising it critically for important intellectual content; final approval of the version to be published and agreement to be accountable for all aspects of the work. L. Altimier: Critical review of content, suggestions for the draft and final manuscript, and language translation.

ACKNOWLEDGMENTS

The authors are very thankful to Bibiana Chinea Jiménez, PNP, MSc, PhD, for her illustrations in this article and to Susana Rodríguez for her critical review and suggestions

DISCLOSURE

Dr A. Sola is a part-time employee of Masimo (Irvine, Ca), Medical Affairs, Neonatology Education and Research. No funding sources for any of the authors.

REFERENCES

1. Priestley J. Experiments and Observations on different kinds of air. Vol. II, London: Johnson, 1775. Available at: http://www.mtsinai.org/pulmonary/papers/ox-hist/ox-hist1.html.
2. Comroe JH Jr. Retrospectroscope. Insights into medical discovery. Menlo Park, California: Von Gehr Press; 1977. p. 114–9. How to Delay Progress Without Even Trying.
3. Wilson J, Long S, Howard P. Respiration of premature infants. Am J Dis Child 1942;63(6):1080–5.
4. Terry TL. Extreme prematurity and fibroblastic overgrowth of persistent vascular sheath behind each crystalline Lens: I. Preliminary Report. Am J Ophthalmol 1942;25:202–3.
5. Terry TL. Fibroblastic overgrowth of persistent tunica vasculosa lentis in infants born prematurely: II. Report of cases-clinical aspects. Trans Am Ophthalmol Soc 1942;40:262–84.
6. Terry TL. Retrolental fibroplasia. J Pediatr 1946;29(6):770–3.
7. Terry TL. Retrolental fibroplasia. Adv Pediatr 1948;3(1):55–67.
8. Reese AB. Retrolental fibroplasia. Am J Ophthalmol 1948;31(1):95.
9. King MJ. Retrolental fibroplasia: a clinical study of two hundred and thirty-eight cases. Arch Ophthalmol 1950;43:694–711.
10. Wood EH, Chang EY, Beck K, et al. 80 Years of vision: preventing blindness from retinopathy of prematurity. J Perinatol 2021;41:1216–24.
11. Gilbert C, Fielder A, Gordillo L, Quinn G, Semiglia R, et al, International NO-ROP Group. Characteristics of infants with severe retinopathy of prematurity in countries with low, moderate and high levels of development; implications for screening. Pediatrics 2005;11:e518–25.
12. Gilbert C. Retinopathy of prematurity: a global perspective of the epidemics, population of babies at risk and implications for control. Early Hum Dev 2008; 84:77–82.
13. Darlow Brian A, Gilbert C. Retinopathy of prematurity – a world update. Semin Perinatol 2019;43(6):315–6.
14. Karna P, Muttineni J, Angell L, et al. Retinopathy of prematurity and risk factors: a prospective cohort study. BMC Pediatr 2005;5:18.
15. Chang JW. Risk factor analysis for the development and progression of retinopathy of prematurity. PLoS One 2019;14(7):e0219934.
16. Gonski S, Hupp SR, Cotten CM, et al. Risk of development of treated retinopathy of prematurity in very low birth weight infants. J Perinatol 2019;39:1562–8.
17. Bonafiglia E, Gusson E, Longo R, et al. Early and late onset sepsis and retinopathy of prematurity in a cohort of preterm infants. Sci Rep 2022;12:11675.

18. de las Rivas Ramírez N, Luque Aranda G, Rius Díaz F, et al. Risk factors associated with Retinopathy of Prematurity development and progression. Sci Rep 2022;12:21977.

19. The Committee for the Classification of Retinopathy of Prematurity. An international classification of retinopathy of prematurity. Arch Ophthalmol 1984;102:1130–4.

20. The international classification of retinopathy of prematurity revisited. Arch Ophthalmol 2005;123(7):991–9.

21. Chiang MF, Quinn GE, Fielder AR et al . International classification of retinopathy of prematurity, 3rd edition. Ophthalmology. 2021;128(10):e51-e68.

22. Molinari A, Weaver C, Jalali S. Classifying retinopathy of prematurity. Community Eye Health 2017;30(99):55–6.

23. Sankar BK, et al. Retinopathy of prematurity: nursing perspective. J Clin Diagn Res 2021;15(4):LE01–6.

24. Flynn JT, Sola A, Good WV, et al. Screening for retinopathy of prematurity - a problem solved? Pediatrics 1995;95(5):755–7.

25. Deodari A, Darlow BA. Preventing sight-threatening ROP: neonatologist's perspectives. Community Eye Health 2017;30(99):50–2.

26. Katoch D, Dogra M. The role of advocacy and communication in reducing ROP in India. Community Eye Health 2018;31(101):32–4.

27. Silva Juan Carlos, Zin A, Gilbert C. Retinopathy of prematurity prevention, screening and treatment programmes: progress in South America. Semin Perinatol 2019;43(6):348–435.

28. Binenbaum G, Tomlinson LA, de Alba Campomanes AG, et al. Postnatal growth and retinopathy of prematurity (G-ROP) study group. Validation of the postnatal growth and retinopathy of prematurity screening criteria. JAMA Ophthalmol 2020;138(1):31–7.

29. Wheeler D, Dobson V, Chiang MF, et al. Retinopathy of prematurity in infants weighing less than 500 grams at birth enrolled in the early treatment for retinopathy of prematurity study. Ophthalmology 2011;118(6):1145–51.

30. Tsai ASH, Acaba-Berrocal L, Sobhy M, et al. Current management of retinopathy of prematurity. Current treatment options in pediatrics 2022;8:246–61.

31. Early Treatment For Retinopathy Of Prematurity Cooperative Group. Revised indications for the treatment of retinopathy of prematurity: results of the early treatment for retinopathy of prematurity randomized trial. Arch Ophthalmol 2003;121(12):1684–94.

32. Good WV. Early treatment for retinopathy of prematurity Cooperative group. Final results of the early treatment for retinopathy of prematurity (ETROP) randomized trial. Trans Am Ophthalmol Soc 2004;102:233–48 [discussion 248-50].

33. Narnaware SH, Bawankule PK, Raje D. Aggressive posterior retinopathy of prematurity (APROP): LASER as the primary modality of treatment. J Ophthalmic Vis Res 2021;16(3):400–7.

34. Fleck BW, Reynolds JD, Zhu Q, et al, RAINBOW Investigator Group. Time course of retinopathy of prematurity regression and Reactivation after treatment with ranibizumab or laser in the RAINBOW trial. Ophthalmol Retina 2022;6(7):628–37.

35. Sankar MJ, Chandra P. Anti-vascular endothelial growth factor (VEGF) drugs for treatment of retinopathy of prematurity Cochrane. Database Syst Rev 2018;2:CD009734.

36. Pertl L, Steinwender G, Mayer C, et al. A systematic review and meta-analysis on the safety of vascular endothelial growth factor (VEGF) inhibitors for the treatment of retinopathy of prematurity. PLoS One 2015;10(6):e0129383.

37. Sola A, Chow L, Rogido M. Retinopathy of prematurity and oxygen therapy: a changing relationship. An Pediatr 2005;62:48–63.

38. Severinghaus JW. Takuo Aoyagi: discovery of pulse oximetry. Anesth Analg 2007;105(6 Suppl):S1–4.

39. Barker SJ. "Motion-Resistant" pulse oximetry; a comparison of new & old models. Anesth Analg 2002;95(4):967–72.

40. Barker SJ, Tremper KK. Pulse oximetry: applications and limitations. Int Anesthesiol Clin 1987;25(3):155–75.

41. Barker SJ. The effects of motion and hypoxemia upon the accuracy of 20 pulse oximeters in human volunteers. Sleep 2002;24:A406–7.

42. Wischniewski E, Erler T, Avenarius S. Multicenter trial of neonatal pulse oximeter sensor usage: a difference between manufacturers. Anesth Analg 2002; 94(A21):S110.

43. Hay WW, Rodden DJ, Collins SM, et al. Reliability of conventional and new pulse oximetry in neonatal patients. J Perinatol 2002;22:360–6.

44. Sahni R, Gupta A, Ohira-Kist K, et al. Motion resistant pulse oximetry in neonates. Arch Dis Child Fetal Neonatal Ed 2003;88:F505–8.

45. Baquero H, Alviz R, Castillo A, et al. Avoiding hyperoxemia during neonatal resuscitation: time to response of different SpO2 monitors. Acta Paediatr 2011;100(4):515–8.

46. Castillo A, Deulofeut R, Sola A. Prevention of retinopathy of prematurity in preterm infants through changes in clinical practice and SpO2 technology. Acta Paediatr 2011;100(2):188–92.

47. Robertson FA, Hoffman GM. Clinical evaluation of the effects of signal integrity and saturation on data availability and accuracy of Masimo SE and Nelcor N-395 oximeters in children. Anesth Analg 2004;98:617–22.

48. Hummler HD, Englemann A, Pohlandt F, et al. Accuracy of pulse oximetry readings in an animal model of low perfusion caused by emerging pneumonia and sepsis. Intens Care Med 2004;30:709–13.

49. Sola A, Chow L, Rogido M. Pulse oximetry in neonatal care in 2005. A comprehensive state of the art review. An Pediatr 2005;62(3):266–81.

50. Barker SJ, Curry J, Redford D, et al. Measurement of carboxyhemoglobin and methemoglobin by pulse oximetry: a human volunteer study. Anesthesiology 2006;105(5):892–7.

51. Barker SJ, Badal JJ. The measurement of dyshemoglobins and total hemoglobin by pulse oximetry. Curr Opin Anaesthesiol 2008;21(6):805–10.

52. Sola A, et al. Safe oxygen saturation targeting and monitoring in preterm infants: can we avoid hypoxia and hyperoxia. Acta Paediatr 2014;103(10):109–18.

53. Barker SJ, Wilson WW. Racial effects on Masimo pulse oximetry: a laboratory study. J Clin Monit Comput 2023;37(2):567–74.

54. Dawson JA, Kamlin CO, Vento M, et al. Defining the reference range for oxygen saturation for infants after birth. Pediatrics 2010;125(6):e1340–7.

55. Dawson JA, Morley CJ. Monitoring oxygen saturation and heart rate in the early neonatal period. Semin Fetal Neonatal Med 2010;15(4):203–7.

56. Kapadia VS, Lal CV, Kakkilaya V, et al. Impact of the neonatal resuscitation Program-recommended low oxygen strategy on outcomes of infants born preterm. J Pediatr 2017;191:35–41.

57. Rabi Y, Dawson JA. Oxygen therapy and oximetry in the delivery room. Semin Fetal Neonatal Med 2013;18(6):330–5.
58. Kapadia V, Wyckoff MH. Oxygen therapy in the delivery room: what is the right dose? Clin Perinatol 2018;45(2):293–306.
59. Kattwinkel J, et al. Neonatal resuscitation: 2010 American heart association guidelines for cardiopulmonary resuscitation and emergency cardiovascular care. Pediatrics 2010;126(5):e1400–13.
60. Wyckoff MH, Weiner CGM, Neonatal Life Support Collaborators. 2020 International Consensus on Cardiopulmonary resuscitation and emergency Cardiovascular care Science with treatment recommendations. Pediatrics 2021;147(Suppl 1). e2020038505C.
61. Welsford M. International Liaison Committee on resuscitation neonatal life support Task Force. Initial oxygen Use for preterm newborn resuscitation: a Systematic review with meta-analysis. Pediatrics 2019;143(1). e20181828.
62. Kapadia VS, Chalak LF, Sparks JE, et al. Resuscitation of preterm neonates with limited versus high oxygen strategy. Pediatrics 2013;132(6):e1488–96.
63. Wyckoff MH and the International Liaison Committee on Resuscitation. 2022 International Consensus on Cardiopulmonary resuscitation and emergency Cardiovascular care Science with treatment recommendations: summary from the basic life support; advanced life support; pediatric life support; neonatal life support; education, implementation, and teams; and first Aid Task Forces. Pediatrics 2023;151(2). e2022060463.
64. Dawson JA, Kamlin CO, Wong C, et al. Oxygen saturation and heart rate during delivery room resuscitation of infants <30 weeks' gestation with air or 100% oxygen. Arch Dis Child Fetal Neonatal Ed 2009;94(2):F87–91.
65. White LN, Thio M, Owen LS, et al. Achievement of saturation targets in preterm infants <32 weeks' gestational age in the delivery room. Arch Dis Child Fetal Neonatal Ed 2017;102(5):F423–7.
66. Dawson JA, Davis PG, O'Donnell CP, et al. Pulse oximetry for monitoring infants in the delivery room: a review. Arch Dis Child Fetal Neonatal Ed 2007; 92(1):F4–7.
67. Saugstad OD, Ramji S, Vento M. Resuscitation of depressed newborn infants with ambient air or pure oxygen: a meta-analysis. Biol Neonate 2005;87:27–34.
68. Saugstad OD, Ramji S, Vento M. Oxygen for newborn resuscitation: how much is enough? Pediatrics 2006;118:789–92.
69. Sola A, Deulofeut R, Rogido M. Oxygen and oxygenation in the delivery room. J Pediatr 2006;148:564–5.
70. Rabi Y, Yee W, Chen SY, et al. Oxygen saturation trends immediately after birth. J Pediatr 2006;148:590–4.
71. Vento M, Saugstad OD. Targeting oxygen in term and preterm infants starting at birth. Clin Perinatol 2019;46(3):459–73.
72. Oei JL, Vento M, Rabi Y, et al. Higher or lower oxygen for delivery room resuscitation of preterm infants below 28 completed weeks gestation: a meta-analysis. Arch Dis Child Fetal Neonatal 2017;102(1):F24–30.
73. O'Donnell CP, Kamlin CO, Davis PG, et al. Clinical assessment of infant colour at delivery. Arch Dis Child Fetal Neonatal Ed 2007;92(6):F465–7.
74. Kamlin CO, O'Donnell CP, Davis PG, et al. Oxygen saturation in healthy infants immediately after birth. J Pediatr 2006;148(5):585–9.
75. Dawson JA, Ekström A, Frisk C, et al. Assessing the tongue colour of newly born infants may help to predict the need for supplemental oxygen in the delivery room. Acta Paediatr 2015;104(4):356–9.

76. Chow LC, Wright KW, Sola A. Can changes in clinical practice decrease the incidence of severe retinopathy of Prematurity in Very Low Birth Weight Infants? Pediatrics 2003;111(2):339–45.

77. York JR, Landers S, Kirby RS, et al. Arterial oxygen fluctuation and retinopathy of prematurity in very-low-birth-weight infants. J Perinatol 2004;24:82–7.

78. Das A, Mhanna M, Sears J, et al. Effect of fluctuation of oxygenation and time spent in the target range on retinopathy of prematurity in extremely low birth weight infants. J Neonatal Perinatal Med 2018;11(3):257–63.

79. Bouzas L, Manzitti J, Sola A, et al. Retinopathy of prematurity in the XXI century in a developing country: an emergency that should be resolved. An Pediatr 2007;66(6):551–8.

80. Gantz MG, SUPPORT Study Group of the Eunice Kennedy Shriver National Institute of Child Health and Human Development Neonatal Research Network. Achieved oxygen saturations and retinopathy of prematurity in extreme preterms. Arch Dis Child Fetal Neonatal Ed 2020;105(2):138–44.

81. Sola A, Zuluaga C. Oxygen saturation targets and retinopathy of prematurity. J AAPOS 2013;17(6):650–2.

82. Sola A. Oxygen saturation in the newborn and the importance of avoiding hyperoxia-induced damage. NeoReviews 2015;16(7):e393.

83. Sola A. Oxygen in neonatal anesthesia: friend or foe? Curr Opin Anaesthesiol 2008;21:332–9.

84. Deulofeut R, Critz A, Adams-Chapman I, et al. Avoiding hyperoxia in infants <1250 g is associated with improved short- and long-term outcomes. J Perinatol 2006;26:700–5.

85. Castillo A, Sola A, Baquero H, et al. Pulse oxygen saturation levels and arterial oxygen tension values in newborns receiving oxygen therapy in the neonatal intensive care Unit: is 85% to 93% an acceptable range? Pediatrics 2008; 121(5):882–9.

86. Deulofeut R, Dudell G, Sola A. Treatment -by- gender effect when aiming to avoid hyperoxia in preterm infants in the NICU. Acta Paediatr 2007;96(7):990–4.

87. Fleck BW, Stenson BJ. Retinopathy of prematurity and the oxygen conundrum: lessons learned from recent randomized trials. Clin Perinatol 2013 Jun;40(2): 229–40.

88. Shukla A, Sonnie C, Sarah W, et al. Comparison of biphasic vs static oxygen saturation targets among infants with retinopathy of prematurity. JAMA Ophthalmol 2019;137(4):417–23.

89. Darlow BA, International Network for Evaluating Outcomes (iNeo) of Neonates. Variations in oxygen saturation targeting, and retinopathy of prematurity screening and treatment criteria in neonatal intensive care Units: an international Survey. Neonatology 2018;114(4):323–31.

90. Askie LM, Darlow BA, Finer N, et al, NeOProM Collaboration. Association between oxygen saturation targeting and death or disability in extremely preterm infants in the neonatal oxygenation prospective meta-analysis Collaboration. JAMA 2018;319(21):2190–201.

91. Bizarro MJ, Li FY, Katz K, et al. Temporal quantification of oxygen saturation ranges: an effort to reduce hyperoxia in the neonatal intensive care unit. J Perinatol 2014;34:33–8.

92. Bizarro MJ. Optimizing oxygen saturation targets in extremely preterm infants. JAMA 2018;319(21):2173–4.

93. Liu T, Tomlinson LA, Yu Y, et al. Changes in institutional oxygen saturation targets are associated with an increased rate of severe retinopathy of prematurity. J AAPOS 2022;26:18.e1–6.
94. Durrani NUR, Karayil Mohammad Ali S, Ede G, et al. Effect of optimizing oxygen saturation targets on the incidence of retinopathy of prematurity in a quaternary NICU. Biomed Hub 2022;7(3):146–55.
95. Aly H, Othman HF, Munster C, et al. The U.S. National trend for retinopathy of prematurity. Am J Perinatol 2022;29(14):1569–76.
96. Klevebro S, Hammar U, Holmström G, et al. Adherence to oxygen saturation targets increased in preterm infants when a higher target range and tighter alarm limits were introduced. Acta Paediatr 2019;108(9):1584–9.
97. Moreton RBR, Fleck BW, Fielder AR, et al. The effect of oxygen saturation targeting on retinal blood vessel growth using retinal image data from the BOOST-II UK Trial. Eye 2016;30:577–81.
98. Perrone S, Giordano M, De Bernardo G, et al. Management of oxygen saturation monitoring in preterm newborns in the NICU: the Italian picture. Ital J Pediatr 2021;47:104.
99. Kang HG, Choi EY, Cho H, et al. Oxygen care and treatment of retinopathy of prematurity in ocular and neurological prognosis. Sci Rep. 2022;12(1):341 www.nature.com/scientificreports/.
100. Hellström A, Smith LEH, Dammann O. Retinopathy of prematurity. Lancet 2013; 382(9902):1445–57.
101. Sola A, Golombek S, Montes Bueno MT, et al. Safe SpO2 targeting and monitoring in preterm infants. How to avoid hypoxia and hyperoxia? Acta Paediatr 2014;103:164–80.
102. Hellström A, Hård AL, Smith LEH. Retinopathy of prematurity. JAMA Ophthalmol 2019;137(4):423–4.
103. Sola A, Chow L. Oxygenation, oxygen saturation, retinopathy of prematurity and other hyperoxia related damage in newborn infants: a return to the basics. In: Govindaswami Balaji, editor. Preventive newborn health and care. Edition 1/e. New Delhi India: Jaypee medical publishers; 2021. 9789352704736.
104. Stenson BJ. Achieved oxygenation saturations and outcome in extremely preterm infants. Clin Perinatol 2019;46:601–10.
105. Claure N, Gerhardt T, Everett R, et al. Closed-loop controlled inspired oxygen concentration for mechanically ventilated very low birth weight infants with frequent episodes of hypoxemia. Pediatrics 2001;107:1120–4.
106. Claure N, Bancalari E, D'Ugard C, et al. Multicenter crossover study of automated control of inspired oxygen in ventilated preterm infants. Pediatrics 2011;127:e76–83.
107. Zapata J, Gómez JJ, Matiz Rubio A, et al. A randomized controlled trial of automated oxygen delivery in preterm neonates receiving supplemental oxygen without mechanical ventilation. Acta Paediatr 2014;101:69–75.
108. Dargaville PA, Marshall AP, McLeod L, et al. Automation of oxygen titration in preterm infants: current evidence and future challenges. Early Hum Dev 2021; 162:105462.
109. Dijkman KP, Mohns T, Dieleman JP, et al. Predictive intelligent control of oxygenation (PRICO) in preterm infants on high flow nasal cannula support: a randomised cross-over study. Arch Dis Child Fetal Neonatal Ed 2021;106:621–6.
110. Dargaville PA, Marshall AP, Ladlow OJ, et al. Automated control of oxygen titration in preterm infants on non-invasive respiratory support. Arch Dis Child Fetal Neonatal Ed 2022;107:39–44.

111. Nair V, Loganathan P, Lal MK, et al. Automated oxygen delivery in neonatal intensive care. Front. Pediatr 2022;10:915312. https://doi.org/10.3389/fped.2022.915312.

112. Sola A. Oxygen management: concerns about both hyperoxia and hypoxia in neonates during critical care and Intraoperatively. In: McCann Mary Ellen, editor. Essentials of anesthesia for infants and neonates. Cambridge University Press; 2019.

113. Sola A and Golombek S. Oxygen saturation in the neonatal period; in Neonatology, Springer International. Editors G Buonocore, et al. DOI 1007/9783319185922911.

114. Kayton A, Timoney P, Vargo L, et al. A review of oxygen physiology and appropriate management of oxygen levels in premature neonates. Adv Neonatal Care 2018;18(2):98–104.

115. Falsaperla R, Giacchi V, Marco Saporito, et al. Pulse oximetry saturation (SpO$_2$) monitoring in the neonatal intensive care Unit (NICU): the challenge for providers. A Systematic review. Adv Neonatal Care 2022;22(3):231–8.

116. Samaja M, Ottolenghi S. The oxygen Cascade from atmosphere to mitochondria as a Tool to understand the (Mal)adaptation to hypoxia. Int J Mol Sci 2023;24(4):3670.

117. Poole DC, Musch TI, Colburn TD. Oxygen flux from capillary to mitochondria: integration of contemporary discoveries. Eur J Appl Physiol 2022;122(1):7–28.

118. Comroe JH Jr, Bahnson ER, Coates EO Jr. Mental changes occurring in chronically anoxemic patients during oxygen therapy. J Am Med Assoc 1950;143:1044–8.

119. Vento M, Asensi M, Sastre J, et al. Resuscitation with room air instead of 100% oxygen prevents oxidative stress in moderately asphyxiated term infants. Pediatrics 2001;107:642–7.

120. Temesvari P, Karg E, Bodi I, et al. Impaired early neurologic outcome in newborn piglets reoxygenated with 100% oxygen compared with room air after pneumothorax-induced asphyxia. Pediatr Res 2001;49:812–9.

121. Wei Yau-Huei, Lee Hsin-Chen. Oxidative stress, mitochondrial DNA mutation, and impairment of antioxidant enzymes in aging. Exp Biol Med 2002;227:671–82.

122. Sola A, Saldeño YP, Favareto V. Clinical practices in neonatal oxygenation: where have we failed? what can we do? J Perinatol 2008;28(1):S28–34.

123. Naumburg E, Bellocco R, Cnattingius S, et al. Supplementary oxygen and risk of childhood lymphatic leukaemia. Acta Paediatr 2002;91:1328–33.

124. Saugstad OD. Oxygen toxicity at birth: the pieces are put together. Pediatr Res 2003;54:789.

125. Felderhoff-Mueser U, Bittigau P, Sifringer M, et al. Oxygen causes cell death in the developing brain. Neurobiol Dis 2004;17:273–82.

126. Shimabuku R, Ota A, Pereyra S, et al. Hyperoxia with 100% oxygen following hypoxia- ischemia increases brain damage in newborn rats. Biol Neonate 2005;88:168–71.

127. Spector LG, Klebanoff MA, Feusner JH, et al. Childhood cancer following neonatal oxygen supplementation. J Pediatr 2005;147:27–31.

128. Paneth N. The evidence mounts against use of pure oxygen in newborn resuscitation. J Pediatr 2005;147:4–6.

129. Sola A, Rogido MR, Deulofeut R. Oxygen as a neonatal health hazard: call for détente in clinical practice. Acta Paediatr 2007;96:801–12.

130. Sola A. Turn off the lights and the oxygen, when not needed: phototherapy and oxidative stress in the neonate. J Pediatr 2007;83(4):293–6.
131. Beharry KD, Cai CL, Valencia GB, et al. Neonatal Intermittent hypoxia, reactive oxygen species, and oxygen-induced retinopathy. React Oxyg Species (Apex) 2017;3(7):12–25.
132. Vento M. Oxidative stress in the perinatal period. Free Radic Biol Med 2019. S0891-5849(19)31232-31238.
133. Perrone S, Lembo C, Gironi F, et al. Erythropoietin as a Neuroprotective drug for newborn infants: Ten Years after the first Use. Antioxidants 2022;11(4):652.
134. Perrone S, Grassi F, Caporilli C, et al. Brain damage in preterm and full-term neonates: serum Biomarkers for the early diagnosis and intervention. Antioxidants 2023;12:309.

Pulse Oximetry Screening for Critical Congenital Heart Defects in Newborn Babies

Anurag Girdhar, DCh, DNB, MRCPCH[a],
Andrew K. Ewer, MD, MRCP, FRCPCH[b],*

KEYWORDS

- Newborn • Congenital heart defects • Pulse oximetry • Screening

KEY POINTS

- Pulse oximetry screening (POS) has consistent test accuracy for the detection of critical congenital heart defects and meets the criteria for universal screening.
- International uptake has been encouraging with most high-income countries now recommending POS.
- POS also detects significant non-cardiac conditions particularly if screening takes place within 24 hours.

INTRODUCTION

Congenital heart defects (CHD) are the most common congenital malformations with an incidence of between 4 and 10 per 1000 livebirths.[1,2] The most severe defects—critical CHD (CCHD)—account for between 15% and 25% of CHD (2–3 per 1000 live births)[1,3,4] and remain a major cause of death and significant morbidity, particularly in the first year of life.[2] CCHD are defined as those leading to death or requiring invasive intervention in the first month of life and are typically "duct-dependent defects" meaning that closure of the ductus arteriosus, which occurs after birth, results in acute cardiovascular collapse or death.[5–7] The majority of CCHD are treatable in the newborn period[8] and as collapse can result in worse surgical outcomes and long-term neurologic impairment,[9–14] early diagnosis before such an event is extremely important.[5]

Most high-income countries routinely screen for CHD using a combination of antenatal ultrasound and postnatal physical examination. Antenatal detection allows for parental counseling and optimization of delivery and postnatal management, but detection rates are highly variable both between and within countries, so although

^a Department of Neonatology, Birmingham Women's Hospital NHS Trust, Birmingham, United Kingdom; ^b Institute of Metabolism and Systems Research, College of Medical and Dental Sciences, University of Birmingham, Birmingham, United Kingdom
* Corresponding author. a.k.ewer@bham.ac.uk

Crit Care Nurs Clin N Am 36 (2024) 99–110
https://doi.org/10.1016/j.cnc.2023.09.001
0899-5885/24/© 2023 Elsevier Inc. All rights reserved.

ccnursing.theclinics.com

individual centers may have excellent detection rates, overall, a significant proportion of defects (up to 70%) are missed.[15–18] Postnatal examination—including auscultation for cardiac murmurs, palpation of peripheral pulses, and visual assessment of cyanosis—is also unreliable and may not detect up to 50% of CCHD.[19] Murmurs are often absent in CCHD; the presence of the ductus arteriosus may allow pulses to be detected and visual assessment of mild to moderate cyanosis is extremely difficult, even for experienced clinicians.[20–22]

SCREENING FOR CRITICAL CONGENITAL HEART DEFECTS WITH PULSE OXIMETRY

These drawbacks have led to the exploration of alternative methods for identifying CCHD and in the early 2000s the first pilot studies investigating the use of pulse oximetry (PO) as a potential screening tool were reported from the United States and Europe.[23–25]

PO is a widely-available, simple, rapid, accurate, and non-invasive method of measuring blood oxygen levels (saturations), and the use of PO as a screen for CCHD is based on the rationale that the majority of newborn babies with CCHD will have a degree of hypoxemia, many of which may be clinically undetectable.[5] If babies were screened with PO in the newborn nursery while still asymptomatic, those with lower saturations could be assessed quickly, and further investigations such as echocardiography could be performed to identify CCHD before life-threatening collapse occurs.

In 2007, 8 of these early studies (which screened a total of 35,960 babies) were analyzed in a systematic review.[26] The review highlighted that there were relatively small numbers of patients in each of the studies, and therefore, a low prevalence of CCHD. There were also significant methodological variations between studies. The review concluded that, although the technique showed promising results, more high-quality studies (in much larger cohorts) were needed to define test accuracy precisely before the PO screening (POS) could be recommended for routine practice.

Between 2009 and 2012, the results of 5 large, well-designed European POS studies were published.[27–31] Although they differed in the timing of screening and the criteria for a positive test (see later), they were of sufficient size and quality to allow robust estimates of test accuracy. Each consistently reported a high specificity (the ability of the test to identify a healthy subject) and moderate sensitivity (the ability to detect the condition of interest), which was a significant improvement over the existing screening tests. Indeed, when POS was added to antenatal ultrasound and postnatal examination in these studies, the CCHD detection rate increased to between 92% and 96%.[32] False positive (FP) rates were clinically acceptable (<1%) and additionally, each study identified babies with clinically important non-cardiac conditions, such as congenital pneumonia and pulmonary hypertension, within the FP group. At the same time, the UK PulseOx study[30] also investigated the parental acceptability of POS[33] and its cost effectiveness,[34] concluding that POS was acceptable to parents (even those whose babies had tested false-positive) and that it was cost-effective in the UK setting.

Following on from these studies, a second systematic review and meta-analysis of 13 POS studies (now including almost 230,000 screened babies) was published in 2012.[35] With this increase in the screened cohort, it was possible to calculate, for the first time, robust estimates of test accuracy for POS (sensitivity 76.5%, specificity 99.9% and FP rate 0.14%). The review concluded that POS met the criteria for universal screening.

Between 2012 and 2018, several more POS studies were published, including the largest-ever study, which screened over 120,000 babies in China.[36] Published in the Lancet, this study reported virtually identical test accuracy and an accompanying editorial raised the suggestion that further similar trials were probably unnecessary.[37]

In 2018, a third systematic review of POS was published in the Cochrane Library, reporting data from 21 POS studies which together had screened over 457,000 babies.[38] Test accuracy (sensitivity 78.5%, specificity 99.8%, FP rate 0.23%) was entirely consistent with the 2012 review.[35] The Cochrane review reported that for every 10,000 apparently healthy newborn infants screened, around 6 of them will have CCHD, and POS will correctly identify 5 of these newborn infants with CCHD (but will miss 1 case), and 9994 will not have CCHD. POS will correctly identify 9980 of these (but 14 newborn infants will be investigated for suspected CCHD). Some of these infants may be exposed to unnecessary additional tests and a prolonged hospital stay, but a proportion will have a potentially serious non-cardiac illness.

This review also concluded that current evidence supported the introduction of routine POS for all asymptomatic newborns in the well-baby nursery.

INTERNATIONAL UPTAKE OF PULSE OXIMETRY SCREENING

An increasing number of countries have recommended universal POS for all apparently healthy newborns >34 weeks gestation and have adopted different ways of achieving this, including national screening recommendations, national recommendations by pediatric/cardiology organizations, and consensus of individual local hospital organizations.

In 2005, Switzerland became the first country to adopt routine POS with the recommendation from the Swiss Societies of Neonatology and Pediatric Cardiology.[39]

Following the work leading to the publication of a study from Poland, the Polish Ministry of Health recommended nationwide POS in 2010.[31]

In the United States in 2011, a workgroup was convened (formed from members of the Secretary's Advisory Committee on Heritable Disorders in Newborns and Children, the American Academy of Pediatrics[AAP], the American College of Cardiology Foundation, and the American Heart Association) to discuss POS with the chief investigators of 2 of the European POS studies[28,30] After the meeting, the decision was made to recommend that POS be added to the routine screening panel for newborns.[40] Following this recommendation, POS was introduced on a state-by-state basis, with all states screening by July 2018. An interim analysis performed by the Centers for Disease Control and Prevention in 2017, which examined almost 27 million births, showed that the introduction of POS in individual states reduced mortality from CCHD by 33% compared with states that were yet to introduce screening[41]

The German Society for Neonatology and Pediatric Intensive Care recommended universal POS in 2012[42] and in 2017, POS was introduced into routine neonatal care throughout Germany.[42] In 2014, the Austrian Society for Pediatrics and Adolescent Medicine also recommended routine POS.[43]

Following on from the important studies in Norway[27] and Sweden,[28] the Nordic countries formally recommended POS in 2014.[44]

In 2013, a pan-European workgroup of neonatologists and cardiologists with an interest in POS encouraged greater uptake, the formulation of policy statements by national professional bodies and European societies,[45] and in 2017 published a European consensus statement on POS.[46]

In the same year, the Spanish Neonatal Society,[47] the Canadian Cardiovascular Society and Canadian Pediatric Cardiology Association,[48] and the Ibero-American Society of Neonatology (Sociedad Iberoamericana de Neonatología [SIBEN] representing all of South and Central America)[49] all issued position statements endorsing the routine use of POS.

POS has been considered by the UK National Screening Committee for many years but they have yet to recommend its implementation. In 2020, a national survey of UK hospitals reported that 51% were routinely screening[50] although more recent unpublished data suggest that this has increased to above 75%. A similar proportion of Australian hospitals are also screening,[51] and a 2017 study in New Zealand funded by the NZ Health Research Council has also advocated its routine introduction.[52]

National recommendations are also in place in Ireland, Saudi Arabia, Abu Dhabi, Kuwait, Israel, China, and Sri Lanka.[53]

ALGORITHM VARIATIONS

Although there is a strong consensus that POS identifies asymptomatic babies with CCHD that would otherwise have been missed, the most appropriate screening pathway (algorithm) that should be used is less clear cut.[54]

As previously mentioned, there is a wide variation in the precise algorithm for POS in the reported studies. The main differences can be grouped as follows: (i) site of saturation testing—that is, post-ductal (foot) only measurement *or* pre-ductal (right hand) *and* post-ductal measurements (including the difference between pre-ductal and post-ductal saturations) and (ii) timing of testing that is, before or after 24 hours of age.[54]

Site of Saturation Testing

The earlier pilot studies[26] (described in the introduction) generally used a single post-ductal saturation measurement in contrast to the pre-ductal and post-ductal measurements used in some of the later studies.[35,38] Some authorities have considered post-ductal measurements to be the most appropriate and efficient way of performing the screening algorithm—as it is quicker and easier to perform than the dual measurements. Indeed, the meta-analyses have not identified a difference in sensitivity between the 2 approaches.[35,38] However, detailed analysis of the raw saturation data from infants who had measurements of both saturations has consistently shown that some babies with CCHD would be missed if only post-ductal measurements were performed.[54] This is particularly apparent in coarctation of the aorta, where there is often a difference between pre-ductal and post-ductal saturations, even with otherwise normal saturations. Also, in transposition of great arteries (particularly with associated aortic obstruction), the post-ductal saturation may be normal while pre-ductal saturations are low.[55] However, despite the potential for missing some CCHD, a number of countries (including Germany, Austria, Ireland, and New Zealand) have recommended post-ductal only screening.[43,52] This perhaps relates to its relative simplicity, concerns about workload for screeners, and the possibility of miscalculating the result. Increasingly, however, the majority of national recommendations are for dual site screening.[35,38]

Timing of Screening

Meta-analysis has consistently shown that the FP rate in studies that screened later (after 24 hours of age) is much lower than in those that screened early (within 24 hours).[35,38] As some healthy newborn infants will have transitional circulation in the first few hours which may result in mild transient hypoxemia, this is perhaps not surprising. This increase in the FP rate has led to many countries (including the United States) to adopt a later screening algorithm (**Fig. 1**). While later screening results in fewer FP results (FP rate – 0.47% < 24 hours vs 0.11% > 24 hours),[38] there is good evidence from later screening studies[28,29] that up to 50% of the infants with CCHDs

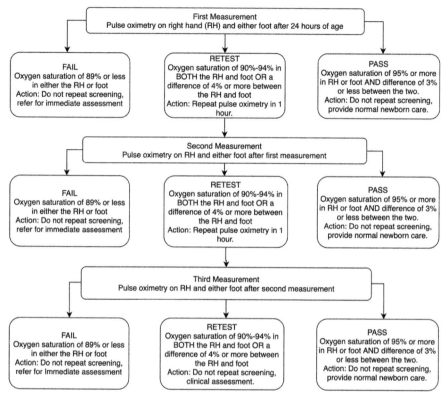

Fig. 1. The US POS algorithm

present with symptoms in the first day of life and around 10% will have pre-diagnosis postnatal collapse,[28] which is the very event that screening aims to prevent. Additionally, early screening is also more likely to detect potentially life-threatening non-cardiac conditions that require early intervention.[56–58] These factors must be considered carefully; although low FPs are important in a screening test, if the majority have a serious non-cardiac condition that requires urgent treatment, this is clearly a significant additional clinical benefit.[56–58] Additionally, postnatal care practices also vary between different countries. In many countries, most otherwise healthy infants are discharged soon after birth, and there are increasing numbers of home births where the midwife leaves the baby a few hours after birth, both making later screening challenging.[58,59]

In the United States, the AAP-recommended algorithm follows that described in a large trial from Sweden[28] where screening took place after 24 hours, measuring pre-ductal and post-ductal oxygen saturations (see **Fig. 1**). The screen is passed if either saturation result is >95% and the difference between the 2 is <3%. A failed screen is either saturation measurement <90%, and a retest is advised if both saturations are between 90% and 95% and/or the difference between the 2 is 4% or more. The algorithm allows for 2 more retests at 1-hour intervals before the test is failed and, referral for further assessment is necessary. This algorithm has also been recommended in Canada.[48]

In the United Kingdom, the majority of screening units[50] have adopted the algorithm described in the UK PulseOx study[30] where babies were screened in the first 24 hours using pre-ductal and post-ductal saturations. The definition of a positive test is slightly different from the US algorithm (**Fig. 2**). With this approach, a positive test is recorded if *either* saturation result is <95% and/or there is a difference of >2%. Any positive test is followed by a clinical assessment. If clinical assessment is abnormal, more detailed assessment is advised. With a normal clinical assessment, a repeat screen is performed after 1 to 2 hours. Using this algorithm in the original study and in subsequent clinical practice, the FP rate was 0.8%.[30,56] However, 79% of the FP cases had significant medical conditions.[56] Only 29% of infants who had a positive test underwent echocardiography, mainly because an alternative non-cardiac diagnosis had been identified. The increased FP rate was mainly due to earlier screening for reasons explained earlier.

In the United States in 2018, an expert workgroup convened a meeting to discuss modifications to the US algorithm and recommended that *both* pre-ductal and post-ductal oxygen saturation should be >95% for a "pass" result and to reduce the repeat screen to only 1 retest in case of an inconclusive test result.[53] Although earlier screening was not recommended, the workgroup agreed that it was acceptable. These recommendations were considered by the AAP, but to date, the recommended algorithm remains unchanged.

Further evidence from the United Kingdom suggests that the performance of the PulseOx algorithm is maintained despite an increase in antenatally-detected CCHD.[60] Over a 6-year period, the proportion of healthy babies admitted to the neonatal unit following a positive test fell from 29% to 2.4% largely as a result of staff confidence in assessing borderline test-positive babies in the well-baby nursery.

FUTURE RESEARCH
Identification of Aortic Obstruction

POS is not a perfect test, and with a sensitivity of 75% - 80%, up to a quarter of babies with CCHD may be missed by POS alone. The commonest defects that are missed are those which lead to aortic obstruction such as coarctation of the aorta (CoA) and interrupted aortic arch. Reported sensitivity for detection of these defects varies but is

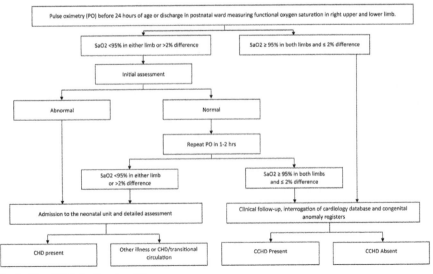

Fig. 2. The UK PulseOx algorithm

usually <50%.[61] Unfortunately, because of the presence of the ductus arteriosus, these are also the most difficult defects to identify by antenatal ultrasound and early clinical assessment. Babies with aortic obstruction are often normoxemic, but there may be differences between pre-ductal and post-ductal saturations, which may be missed by measuring post-ductal saturations only.[54] A more conservative cut-off for the pre/post difference may increase the detection but there are currently insufficient data to support this.[54] National raw saturation data from screening babies with CCHD may help with this but, these data have not been made available.

For a number of years, there has been considerable interest in the use of perfusion index (PI) as a potential additional screen for defects such as CoA. PI is an objective assessment of the peripheral pulse and can be measured by new-generation pulse oximeters at the same time as oxygen saturations. As peripheral perfusion is often compromised in aortic obstruction, the potential usefulness of PI as a screen for these defects is logical. There have been a number of relatively small studies evaluating the test accuracy of PI to detect CCHD with aortic obstruction,[61,62] but to date, the evidence, although promising, is insufficient to recommend PI as a screening test.[61,62] The main difficulties are precise definitions of the normal range in newborn infants and a lack of a consistent, robust cut-off value for a positive test.

Use of Pulse Oximetry Screening in Low-to-middle-income Countries

Most deaths from CHDs occur in low-to-middle-income countries (LMICs), and the proportion is rising as care improves for infectious diseases and malnutrition. While the infant mortality from CHDs has declined by over 50% in richer countries, the decline is only 6% in low-income countries.[2] The World Health Organization has prioritized a reduction in premature deaths from non-communicable diseases, including CHDs. Although resources may not always be available to treat CCHD, POS can also detect babies with non-cardiac conditions such as pneumonia and sepsis. The burden of neonatal sepsis is much higher in LMICs, with neonatal sepsis rates 1.8 times in middle-income countries and 3.5 times in low-income countries when compared to high-income countries.[63] Small feasibility studies in LMIC investigating the potential of POS to detect early-onset neonatal sepsis have shown promising results;[64-66] however, much larger trials are needed to evaluate this appropriately. POS particularly if performed in the first 24 hours, does detect a significant number of neonatal infections, and as treatment requires relatively fewer resources, POS has the potential to reduce neonatal morbidity and mortality in LMICs.

SUMMARY

POS is quick, simple, feasible, cost-effective, acceptable, improves the detection rate for CCHD, and significantly reduces mortality. POS meets the criteria for universal screening and has been adopted into routine postnatal practice in many high-income countries. POS also identifies a significant number of babies with potentially life-threatening non-cardiac conditions, particularly in the first 24 hours of life, which is an important additional benefit.

The most effective screening algorithm is still a subject of debate, but it is important to remember that whichever algorithm is used, all are superior to existing screening methods. Perhaps a balance needs to be struck between detection of serious illness and limiting false-positive results, and local circumstances may play an influence in this respect. More data from larger populations may help to refine the screening algorithm further. Awareness that PO screening is not a perfect test and that babies with CCHD may still be missed, is also very important. Therefore, PO screening should be introduced in addition to existing screening methods and healthcare workers and parents need to be aware of the limitations of the test. Investigation of alternative technologies to identify problematic defects such as CoA should be encouraged.

CLINICS CARE POINTS

- Babies with aortic obstruction e.g. coarctation of the aorta may be missed by all screening methods including PO screening. A high degree of clinical suspicion should remain for babies who have minor symptoms despite negative screens.
- Consideration should be given to the optimum timing for PO screening in different clinical settings.
- Routine collection of PO screening data (ie, raw saturations at screening and clinical outcomes) may support further modification of screening algorithms.

FUNDING

The primary funder was the NIHR through a Health Technology Assessment (HTA) grant.

DISCLOSURE

The authors confirm no financial disclosures or conflicts of interest.

REFERENCES

1. Hoffman JI, Kaplan S. The incidence of congenital heart disease. J Am Coll Cardiol 2002;39(12):1890–900.
2. Zimmerman MS, Smith AGC, Sable CA, et al. Global, regional, and national burden of congenital heart disease, 1990–2017: a systematic analysis for the Global Burden of Disease Study 2017. Lancet Child Adolesc Heal 2020;4(3): 185–200.
3. Bakker MK, Bergman JEH, Krikov S, et al. Prenatal diagnosis and prevalence of critical congenital heart defects: an international retrospective cohort study. BMJ Open 2019;9(7):e028139.
4. Mouledoux JH, Walsh WF. Evaluating the diagnostic gap: statewide incidence of undiagnosed critical congenital heart disease before newborn screening with pulse oximetry. Pediatr Cardiol 2013;34(7):1680–6.
5. Ewer AK, Furmston AT, Middleton LJ, et al. Pulse oximetry as a screening test for congenital heart defects in newborn infants: a test accuracy study with evaluation of acceptability and cost-effectiveness. Health Technol Assess 2012; 16(2):1–184.
6. Mahle WT, Newburger JW, Matherne GP, et al. Role of pulse oximetry in examining newborns for congenital heart disease: a scientific statement from the American Heart Association and American Academy of Pediatrics. Circulation 2009; 120(5):447–58.
7. Hoffman JIE. It is time for routine neonatal screening by pulse oximetry. Neonatology 2011;99:1–9.
8. Bruno CJ, Havranek T. Screening for critical congenital heart disease in newborns. Adv Pediatr 2015;62(1):211–26.

9. Brown KL, Ridout DA, Hoskote A, et al. Delayed diagnosis of congenital heart disease worsens preoperative condition and outcome of surgery in neonates. Heart 2006;92(9):1298–302.

10. CLv Velzen, Haak MC, Reijnders G, et al. Prenatal detection of transposition of the great arteries reduces mortality and morbidity. Ultrasound Obstet Gynecol 2015; 45:320–5.

11. Limperopoulos C, Majnemer A, Shevell MI, et al. Predictors of developmental disabilities after open heart surgery in young children with congenital heart defects. J Pediatr 2002;141:51–8.

12. Mahle WT, Tavani F, Zimmerman RA, et al. An MRI study of neurological injury before and after congenital heart surgery. Circulation 2002;106(12 Suppl 1): I109–14.

13. Bonnet D, Coltri A, Butera G, et al. Detection of transposition of the great arteries in fetuses reduces neonatal morbidity and mortality. Circulation 1999;99(7): 916–8.

14. Fixler DE, Xu P, Nembhard WN, et al. Age at referral and mortality from critical congenital heart disease. Pediatrics 2014;134:e98–105.

15. Quartermain MD, Pasquali SK, Hill KD, et al. Variation in prenatal diagnosis of congenital heart disease in infants. Pediatrics 2015;136:e378–85.

16. Sharland G. Fetal cardiac screening and variation in prenatal detection rates of congenital heart disease: why bother with screening at all? Future Cardiol 2012;8(2):189–202.

17. National congenital Heart disease Audit 2019 summary report (2017/18 data). https://www.hqip.org.uk/wp-content/uploads/2019/09/Ref-129-Cardiac-NCHDA-Summary-Report-2019-FINAL.pdf.

18. Corcoran S, Briggs K, H OC, et al. Prenatal detection of major congenital heart disease - optimising resources to improve outcomes. Eur J Obstet Gynecol Reprod Biol 2016;203:260–3.

19. Wren C, Richmond S, Donaldson L. Presentation of congenital heart disease in infancy: implications for routine examination. Arch Dis Child Fetal Neonatal 1999;80:F49–53.

20. Ainsworth SB, Wyllie JP, Wren C. Prevalence and clinical significance of cardiac murmurs in neonates. Arch Dis Child Fetal Neonatal 1999;80:F43–5.

21. Gaskin PR, Owens SE, Talner NS, et al. Clinical auscultation skills in pediatric residents. Pediatrics 2000;105(6):1184–7.

22. O'Donnell CPF, Kamlin COF, Davis PG, et al. Clinical assessment of infant colour at delivery. Arch Dis Child Fetal Neonatal Ed 2007;92:F465–7.

23. Richmond S, Reay G, Abu Harb M. Routine pulse oximetry in the asymptomatic newborn. Arch Dis Child Fetal Neonatal Ed 2002;87(2):F83–8.

24. Koppel RI, Druschel CM, Carter T, et al. Effectiveness of pulse oximetry screening for congenital heart disease in asymptomatic newborns. Pediatrics 2003;111(3): 451–5.

25. Sendelbach DM, Jackson GL, Lai SS, et al. Pulse oximetry screening at 4 hours of age to detect critical congenital heart defects. Pediatrics 2008;122(4):e815–20.

26. Thangaratinam S, Daniels J, Ewer AK, et al. The accuracy of pulse oximetry in screening for congenital heart disease in asymptomatic newborns: a systematic review. Arch Dis Child Fetal Neonatal Ed 2007;92:F176–80.

27. Meberg A, Brügmann-Pieper S, Due R Jr, et al. First day of life pulse oximetry screening to detect congenital heart defects. J Pediatr 2008;152(6):761–5.

28. de-Wahl Granelli A, Wennergren M, Sandberg K, et al. Impact of pulse oximetry screening on the detection of duct dependent congenital heart disease: a Swedish prospective screening study in 39,821 newborns. BMJ 2009;338:a3037.
29. Riede FT, Wörner C, Dähnert I, et al. Effectiveness of neonatal pulse oximetry screening for detection of critical congenital heart disease in daily clinical routine–results from a prospective multicenter study. Eur J Pediatr 2010;169(8):975–81.
30. Ewer AK, Middleton LJ, Furmston AT, et al, PulseOx Study Group. Pulse oximetry screening for congenital heart defects in newborn infants (PulseOx): a test accuracy study. Lancet 2011;378(9793):785–94.
31. Turska Kmieć A, Borszewska Kornacka MK, Błaż W, et al. Early screening for critical congenital heart defects in asymptomatic newborns in Mazovia province: experience of the POLKARD pulse oximetry programme 2006-2008 in Poland. Kardiol Pol 2012;70(4):370–6.
32. Ewer AK. Review of pulse oximetry screening for critical congenital heart defects in newborn infants. Current Opinion in Cardiology 2013;92–6.
33. Powell R, Pattison HM, Bhoyar A, et al. Pulse oximetry as a screening test for congenital heart defects in newborn infants: an evaluation of acceptability to mothers. Arch Dis Child Fetal Neonatal Ed 2012;98:F59–63.
34. Roberts TE, Barton P, Auguste P, et al. Pulse oximetry as a screening test for congenital heart disease in newborn infants: a cost effectiveness analysis. Arch Dis Child 2012;97:221–6.
35. Thangaratinam S, Brown K, Zamora J, et al. Pulse oximetry screening for critical congenital heart defects in asymptomatic newborn babies: a systematic review and meta-analysis. Lancet 2012;379(9835):2459–64.
36. Zhao QM, Ma XJ, Ge XL, et al, Neonatal Congenital Heart Disease screening group. Pulse oximetry with clinical assessment to screen for congenital heart disease in neonates in China: a prospective study. Lancet 2014;384(9945):747–54.
37. Ewer AK. Pulse oximetry screening: do we have enough evidence now? Lancet 2014;384:725–6.
38. Plana MN, Zamora J, Suresh G, et al. Pulse oximetry screening for critical congenital heart defects. Cochrane Database Syst Rev 2018;3(3):Cd011912.
39. Arlettaz R, Bauersfeld U. Recommandations concernant le screening néonatal des cardiopathies congénitales. Pediatrica 2005;16(5):38–41.
40. Kemper AR, Mahle WT, Martin GR, et al. Strategies for implementing screening for critical congenital heart disease. Pediatrics 2011;128(5):e1259–e1267.
41. Abouk R, Grosse SD, Ailes EC, et al. Association of US state implementation of newborn screening policies for critical congenital heart disease with early infant cardiac deaths. JAMA 2017;2111–8.
42. Riede F-T, Paech C, Orlikowsky T. Pulse oximetry screening in Germany-historical aspects and future perspectives. Int J Neonatal Screen 2018;4(2):15.
43. Fritz M, Fritsch P, Foramitti M, et al. Pulse Oximetries Screening bei Neugeborenen auf kritische angeborene Herzfehler. Monatsschr Kinderheilkd 2014;162(7):638–43.
44. de-Wahl Granelli A, Meberg A, Ojala T, et al. Nordic pulse oximetry screening–implementation status and proposal for uniform guidelines. Acta Paediatr 2014;103(11):1136–42.
45. Ewer AK, Granelli AD, Manzoni P, et al. Pulse oximetry screening for congenital heart defects. Lancet 2013;382(9895):856–7.
46. Manzoni P, Martin GR, Sanchez Luna M, et al, European Pulse Oximetry Screening Workgroup. Pulse oximetry screening for critical congenital heart

defects: a European consensus statement. Lancet Child Adolesc Health 2017; 1(2):88–90.

47. Sánchez Luna M, Pérez Muñuzuri A, Sanz López E, et al. [Pulse oximetry screening of critical congenital heart defects in the neonatal period. The Spanish National Neonatal Society recommendation]. An Pediatr 2018;88(2):112, e1-.e6.

48. Wong KK, Fournier A, Fruitman DS, et al. Canadian cardiovascular society/Canadian pediatric cardiology association position statement on pulse oximetry screening in newborns to enhance detection of critical congenital heart disease. Can J Cardiol 2017;33:199–208.

49. Sola A, Golombek SG. Early detection with pulse oximetry of hypoxemic neonatal conditions. Development of the IX clinical consensus statement of the Ibero-American society of Neonatology (SIBEN). Int J Neonatal Screen 2018;4(1):10.

50. Brown S, Liyanage S, Mikrou P, et al. Newborn pulse oximetry screening in the UK: a 2020 survey. Lancet 2020;396(10255):881.

51. Kluckow M. Barriers to the implementation of newborn pulse oximetry screening: a different perspective. Int J Neonatal Screen 2018;4(1):4.

52. Cloete E, Gentles TL, Alsweiler JM, et al. Should New Zealand introduce nationwide pulse oximetry screening for the detection of critical congenital heart disease in newborn infants? N Z Med J 2017;130(1448):64–9.

53. Martin GR, Ewer AK, Gaviglio A, et al. Updated strategies for pulse oximetry screening for critical congenital heart disease. Pediatrics 2020;146(1): e20191650.

54. Ewer AK, Martin GR. Newborn pulse oximetry screening: which algorithm is best? Pediatrics 2016;138:e20161206.

55. Yap SH, Anania N, Alboliras ET, et al. Reversed differential cyanosis in the newborn: a clinical finding in the supracardiac total anomalous pulmonary venous connection. Pediatr Cardiol 2009;30(3):359–62.

56. Singh A, Rasiah SV, Ewer AK. The impact of routine predischarge pulse oximetry screening in a regional neonatal unit. Arch Dis Child Fetal Neonatal Ed 2014; 99(4):F297–302.

57. Ward J, Motwani J, Baker N, et al. Congenital methemoglobinemia identified by pulse oximetry screening. Pediatrics 2019;143:e20182814.

58. Narayen IC, Blom NA, Verhart MS, et al. Adapted protocol for pulse oximetry screening for congenital heart defects in a country with homebirths. Eur J Pediatr 2015;174(1):129–32.

59. Cawsey MJ, Noble S, Cross-Sudworth F, et al. Feasibility of pulse oximetry screening for critical congenital heart defects in homebirths. Arch Dis Child Fetal Neonatal Ed 2016. https://doi.org/10.1136/archdischild-2015-309936.

60. Henderson A, Aguirre D, Singh A, et al. Temporal trends in routine predischarge pulse oximetry screening: 6 years' experience in a UK regional neonatal unit. Arch Dis Child - Fetal and Neonatal Edition 2022;107:256–61.

61. Ewer AK. Perfusion index as a screening test for neonatal aortic coarctation: should we be using it routinely? Acta Paediatr 2021;110:1716–7.

62. Ewer AK. Perfusion index cannot be currently recommended as an additional newborn screen for critical congenital heart disease: more data needed. Arch Dis Child 2019;104:411–2.

63. Popescu CR, Cavanagh MMM, Tembo B, et al. Neonatal sepsis in low-income countries: epidemiology, diagnosis and prevention. Expert Rev Anti Infect Ther 2020;18(5):443–52.

64. King EM, Lieu C, Kasasa A, et al. Pulse oximetry as a screening tool to detect hypoxia associated with early-onset sepsis in asymptomatic newborns: a feasibility study in a low-income country. JAMMR 2013;4(5):1115–28.

65. Swamy R, Razak A, Mohanty P, et al. Pulse oximetry as screening test for early-onset sepsis in newborns in tertiary hospitals in India. Journal of Neonatology 2015;29(4):1–3.

66. Jones AJ, Howarth C, Nicholl R, Mat-Ali E, Knowles R. The impact and efficacy of routine pulse oximetry screening for CHD in a local hospital. Cardiol Young 2016; 26(7):1397–405.

Midline Catheter Use in the Neonatal Intensive Care Unit

Stephanie Sykes, DNP, APRN-CNP, NNP-BC*,
Jodi Ulloa, DNP, APRN-CNP, NNP-BC, Deborah Steward, PhD, RN

KEYWORDS

- Vascular access devices • Midline catheters • Neonatal • Clinical guidelines

KEY POINTS

- Vascular access is critical to the management of acutely/critically ill neonates.
- Maintaining vascular access in acutely/critically ill neonates is difficult due to vascular immaturity and fragility and flexibility of subcutaneous tissue.
- Multiple, painful peripheral intravenous catheter insertions can negatively impact neurodevelopment in acutely/critically ill neonates, especially those born preterm.
- Midline catheters offer a solution between peripheral intravenous catheters and peripherally inserted central catheters due to fewer complications, fewer insertion attempts, and longer dwell times.

INTRODUCTION

Neonates admitted to the neonatal intensive care unit (NICU) are a unique population who most often begin life acutely or critically ill. The NICU population is characterized by a large range of gestational ages, variability in the appropriateness of birthweight for gestational age, and cohorts of neonates confronting unique illnesses due to preterm birth.[1] Venous access is required by most acutely/critically ill neonates, especially those born preterm. Access is required for implementing management strategies such as stabilization, medications, fluids, nutrition, and transfusion of blood products. However, achieving and maintaining venous access in these neonates can be difficult, especially in preterm infants. Their veins are small and fragile, coupled with physiologic immaturity that increases the risk of venous/capillary leakage.[2–4] In addition, the subcutaneous tissue is flexible, allowing for easy expansion with fluid from vascular leakage.[4] Many neonates may require vascular access for weeks or months, putting the neonate at risk for multiple attempts to obtain vascular access across time as well as complications.

Peripheral intravenous (PIV) catheters and peripherally inserted central catheters (PICC) are 2 common vascular access approaches used in the NICU and have

The Ohio State University College of Nursing, 295 West 10th Avenue, Columbus, OH 43210, USA
* Corresponding author.
E-mail address: sykes.129@osu.edu

Crit Care Nurs Clin N Am 36 (2024) 111–118
https://doi.org/10.1016/j.cnc.2023.09.004
ccnursing.theclinics.com

traditionally been the most studied in the neonatal literature. PICCs offer a long-term solution for venous access in neonates due to their central placement and allow for the infusion of nutritional products, fluids, and medications that can be difficult on peripherally located veins due to fluid pH, osmolarity, or cytotoxicity.[2] PIVs are intended for short-term needs and prove to be a challenge in accessing and maintaining. Both options offer advantages and disadvantages. An alternative to PIVs and PICCs is the midline peripheral catheter (MPC), which in the literature may also be referred to as an extended dwell peripheral intravenous catheter. Depending on the intended use, the MPC offers a venous access approach between a PIV and a PICC.[5] Usage of MPCs in the NICU is slowly increasing with the limited published evidence suggesting they are viable options when considering the need for vascular access.[1,6] The purpose of this article is to present the advantages and disadvantages of MPCs as an alternative approach for venous access in neonates when appropriate.

Definitions: Common Vascular Access Devices

Reliance on PIVs and PICCs is common and a life-sustaining practice in the NICU. Intended use, as well as advantages and disadvantages, are associated with both approaches. PIV catheters are venous catheters short in length[7] and widely used in the NICU for both emergent and non-emergent situations. Common usage sites include the hand, forearm, foot, and scalp. Their suggested use includes infusion of non-vesicant fluids such as $\leq$ 12.5% dextrose, total parenteral nutrition with osmolarity $\leq$ 900 mOsm/L, medications, and blood therapy.[8] Unfortunately, PIVs are difficult to successfully place on first attempt, often requiring multiple attempts for access. Legemaat and colleagues[9] reported a first-attempt success rate of 45% with neonates enduring, on average, 2.22 attempts. In addition to the risk of multiple attempts, the other issue is dwell time once successfully inserted. A PIV is not recommended for prolonged dwell times with a limited duration of <4 days as the suggested target.[7] However, reported dwell times in neonates have been found to be approximately 48 hours, often requiring reinsertion of a PIV.[9]

Small PIV catheters are difficult to maintain and vulnerable to numerous complications. The complication rate of PIVs in neonates has been reported to be at least 50%[2] with reports as high as 63%.[10] Infiltration/extravasation is the most reported complication. Rates of infiltration/extravasation are reported to occur in greater than 60% of neonates, with immaturity as a significant risk factor.[2,9,11] Unfortunately, rates of infiltration and extravasation are reported together. However, fluids characterized as highly acidic or alkalotic, having a higher osmolarity, or more vasoactive or cytotoxic are more often associated with extravasation.[2] Because of immaturity of their skin and fragility of their small veins, preterm infants are at higher risk for skin damage and extravasation injuries.[12-14] Other reported complications include phlebitis, catheter occlusion, and infection, which has increased risk after > 72 hours of placement if blood remains in the hub.[10] Infiltration and infection of PIV catheters have been identified among the most common preventable safety events that occur in NICUs.[15]

An important issue associated with complications is the non-elective removal of the catheter, with rates paralleling the complication rate.[9] Non-elective removal results in subjecting the neonate to further stress and painful catheter placement attempts. Legemaat and colleagues[9] reported that the placement of 62% of catheters resulted from a complication with a previous catheter. The potential consequences of multiple attempts are not benign as it is well documented that early painful experiences, especially in preterm infants, can negatively impact neurodevelopment.[16]

PICCs are an important component of NICU care, allowing for long-term venous access. The targeted placement goal for the tip of a PICC line is to centrally locate it in either the superior vena cava (SVC) or the inferior vena cava (IVC). Catheters inserted via the upper arm and scalp are threaded to the SVC and from the lower extremity into the IVC.[17] The most common veins used in neonates include the basilic, cephalic, axillary, great saphenous, popliteal, and temporal and posterior auricular veins in the scalp.[18] However, central placement can be difficult in some neonates due to small vein diameters, obstructing valves in the vein, or venous tortuosity.[19]

There are several advantages associated with the use of PICCs in neonates. These catheters can be inserted and removed without anesthesia.[20] They allow for the infusion of vasoactive or continuous medications, long courses of antibiotics, hyperosmolar fluids, and calorically dense parenteral nutrition, especially to preterm infants whose gastrointestinal tract is developmentally immature and unable to tolerate enteral nutrition.o[21] In addition, successful PICC placement decreases the number of painful IV attempts, decreasing the neonate's stress exposure.[16]

As with PIVs, complications can occur with the use of PICCs, often resulting in removal and reinsertion of the catheter depending upon the neonate's needs. Complication rates have been reported to range from approximately 20% to 30%.[19,22–24] However, PICCs that are not located centrally have a higher complication rate[19,23,24] and a significantly shorter dwell time.[23] Documented PICC complications include catheter migration,[21] infection,[19,21,22,24] phlebitis,[19,24] occlusion,[21,22,24] infiltration,[21,22,24] and catheter leakage.[19]

BACKGROUND OF MIDLINE PERIPHERAL CATHETERS

MPCs are increasingly being recognized for their beneficial use in neonates as the technology of MPCs (ie, catheter material) continues to evolve.[1,6] The MPCs are longer in length than PIVs and are more durable than PIVs.[25] They offer an alternative to usual vascular access devices for neonates who require venous access for greater than 3 days but do not require prolonged access.[3] Given the difficulties in maintaining PIVs in neonates, the rationale behind their use in neonates is to improve dwell time, maintain uninterrupted IV therapy, limit the number of venipunctures, allow access for obtaining blood for labs, and decrease the number of complications associated with vascular access devices, especially PIVs.[5] Thus, the suggested benefits of MPCs make them an attractive option for use with neonates.

MPCs are inserted under sterile conditions. They are inserted into select, deeper peripheral veins, are not threaded to be centrally located, and do not require X-ray confirmation for placement.[26] Peripheral veins commonly selected in neonates are in the upper forearm, lower extremity, and scalp. When threaded, the distal tip for forearm veins should be located at or below the axillary vein, below the inguinal fold for the lower extremity, and jugular vein above the clavicle for a scalp vein.[7] In neonates, midline catheters are usually 8 cm or 15 cm in length with the selected length based on the size of the infant.[27] It is recommended that a small dose of heparin, per unit policy, is a component of infused fluids or a heparin lock is utilized to maintain catheter patency and prevent occlusion.[13,27,28]

Limited published evidence suggests that there are clinical situations where neonates may benefit from the use of an MPC. The growing interest in their appropriate use in neonates is supported by the early, pioneering work with neonates where MPCs were successfully used in the NICU.[28–30] Adding to the growing interest is their successful usage in adults and children. Evaluation of MPCs in a prospective, multicenter study with adult patients found that MPCs were a better choice than a

PICC line to meet the needs for short-term access (<30 days) and had fewer complications.[31] In a comparison with PIVs, MPCs were found to require less catheter insertion attempts, had fewer complications, and improved dwell time.[32] Findings from a randomized feasibility study comparing PIVs with MPCs demonstrated that MPCs resulted in less failed attempts, greater dwell time, and fewer catheter-related complications (Marsh).[33] In addition, findings from a recent systematic review demonstrated that MPCs have a high insertion success rate and are safe and reliable to use in both adults and children. Of note, the MPCs improved the quality of patient care.[34] The reported findings indicate that MPCs serve an important clinical purpose in adults.

Research findings from the use of MPCs with children are of interest to neonatal health care providers since children often experience some of the same issues with PIVs that neonates do, such as shorter dwell time, multiple attempts, and procedural pain and stress.[35] Much of what is known about MPC use in children is based on descriptive research[34] or from children who are chronically ill and require intermittent intravenous medications for illness management, that is, children with cystic fibrosis (CF).[36]

Results from a trial use of MPCs in children demonstrated a high success rate with catheter insertion (>80%) and proved to be a successful alternative to a PICC or PIV for children who required less than 30 days of venous access.[37,38] In one of the only randomized clinical trials with children comparing MPCs to PIVs, MPCs had significantly longer dwell times, fewer failed catheters after placement, and more children were likely to complete their course of treatment with 1 catheter placement.[25] Importantly, both parents and children were more satisfied in the MPC group.

In a second randomized clinical trial, children with CF who required antibiotics for pulmonary optimization were randomly assigned to either a PICC group or a MPC group. Fewer children in the MPC group required general anesthesia for catheter placement. MPCs were associated with a shorter procedure time, fewer catheter placement attempts, and less patient cost.[36] Like the reported satisfaction reported by Qin and colleagues,[25] parents and children in this study reported less anxiety and greater satisfaction with the experience.[36] The available reported evidence suggests that MPC use in children has resulted in positive outcomes and a documented role for MPCs in children. However, findings from a recent systematic review suggest a cautious approach as compelling evidence is needed.[39]

The reported use of MPCs in the NICU began in the 1990s. These catheters were successfully placed in both full-term and preterm neonates.[28,29] Early studies of MPCs demonstrated increased dwell times, fewer venipunctures, and fewer complications when compared to PIVs.[28–30] These early findings were supported by more recent, albeit limited, documentation of successful use of MPCs in the NICU. Chenoweth and colleagues[6] evaluated the introduction of MPCs in their NICU. Their findings indicated that a significant number of placed MPCs remained in place for the duration of intended use, and infiltration was the most common complication (14.9%). Interestingly, the authors noted that missed opportunities for MPC placement could have maximized their use. Evaluation of unit protocol development for the use of MPCs demonstrated longer dwell times, fewer catheter placement attempts, and fewer complications.[1,3]

Findings from the study by Tsunozaki and colleagues[13] are congruent with previously reported findings. Neonates with an MPV catheter experienced longer dwell times, required fewer catheter placements, and had fewer complications. Although the reported evidence is limited, the data indicate neonates may benefit from the use of MPCs during their treatment when appropriate. Experience with the use of

MPCs with institutional protocols in 2 midwestern Level IV NICUs for specific patient populations have been decidedly supportive of their clinical usefulness. The MPCs have been used in these NICUs for long-term antibiotic therapy, blood draws, and IV therapy. While there is variation in the protocols between institutions, the use and complications associated with MPCs are consistent with the evidence in the literature (Personal Communication: Sykes and Ulloa).

As with other venous access devices, there are advantages and disadvantages associated with midline catheter use in neonates. As documented study findings indicate, advantages of PMCs include increased dwell times,[1,3,13] fewer painful venipunctures,[1,3,6,13] and fewer complications.[1,6] In addition, MPCs may provide access for venous access in neonates whose veins prove difficult to access, thus decreasing the number of painful attempts.[1,3,6] These catheters may also be useful in situations where a critically ill neonate has a PICC in place but requires a second venous access device.[3] Because the MPC is placed in a larger vein, the proximal placement in the extremity allows for hemodilution of the intravenous solution and limiting irritation of the vein.[13] Lastly, the catheter softens from body temperature decreasing vein irritation and allowing movement of the extremities.[1]

There are several disadvantages associated with the use of MPCs. Most important are the associated complications. Rates of the types of complications varied among the reported studies. Infiltration is a common complication.[1,3,6] Other complications include dislodgement, occlusion, phlebitis, leakage, thrombus, and infection.[1,3,6,13] While not a significant factor, placement of an MPC requires specifically trained NICU providers, limiting the number of available personnel to place the catheter.[1] While not necessarily a disadvantage, a conundrum is whether to place MPCs in all neonates or limit the usefulness of MPCs to specific gestational age or birthweight categories.

DISCUSSION AND RECOMMENDATIONS

Introduction and acceptance of MPC usage in a specific NICU may require several steps. Units may find it helpful to analyze their data related to PIV and PICC usage to establish a need for the MPCs. Hospital and NICU administrators must be willing to provide the time and resources necessary to train NICU providers, most often nurses, as well as educating the remaining providers.[1] A unit protocol or algorithm should be developed, based on the available evidence, to guide uses and selection of eligible neonates.[1,3,6] Should MPC usage be introduced, gathering data on key variables such as insertion rates, number of attempts, dwell times, and complications will be critical.[1] In addition, feedback from NICU healthcare providers will be important.

SUMMARY

Vascular access is necessary for the successful management of neonates in the NICU. However, selecting and inserting the appropriate vascular access device remains challenging. Further, it is critical that any device inserted limits the harm to the neonate and optimizes treatment.[39] The available but limited, evidence supports the use of MPCs with neonates as, the advantages appear to outweigh the disadvantages. However, more studies, especially randomized clinical trials, are greatly needed in neonatal patients to further develop strong evidence to support their varied use in the NICU, as well as increase their accepted use among neonatal providers.[5,6] An intervention that appears to be beneficial to neonates and includes the potential advantage of a less painful, stress-producing procedure is critical to neonatal neurodevelopment, especially preterm infants.[16]

CLINICS CARE POINTS

- Selection and insertion of appropriate vascular access devices in the NICU can directly influence patient outcomes.
- Evidence to support the use of midline catheters in the NICU is increasing but, more clinical trials are needed to develop practice guidelines.
- New procedures in the NICU, such as the use of MPCs, require appropriate staff training, management strategies, and quality monitoring to track potential complications.

DISCLOSURE

The authors do not have any potential conflicts of interest and do not have any relevant financial and/or nonfinancial relationships to disclose for the publication of this article.

REFERENCES

1. Marchetti JM, Blaine T, Shelly CE, et al. Effective use of extended dwell peripheral intravenous catheters in neonatal intensive care patients. Adv Neonatal Care 2023;23(1):93–101.
2. Danski MTR, Mingorance P, Johann DA, et al. Incidence of local complications and risk factors associated with peripheral intravenous catheter in neonates. Rev Esc Enfrerm USP 2016;50(1):22–8.
3. Romitti MG, Perez CR, Pezzotti E, et al. Long peripheral catheters in neonates: filling the gap between short peripheral catheters and epicutaneous-caval catheters? J Vasc Access 2021;17. 11297298211057377.
4. Wu J, Mu D. Vascular catheter-related complications in newborns. J Paediatr Child Health 2012;48(2):E91–5.
5. Tripathi S, Kuman S, Kaushik S. The practice and complications of midline catheters: a systematic review. Crit Cate Med 2021;49(2):e140–50.
6. Chenoweth KB, Guo J-W, Chan B. The extended dwell peripheral intravenous catheter is an alternative method of NICU intravenous access. Adv Neonatal Care 2018;18(4):295–301.
7. Gorski LA, Hadaway L, Hagle ME, et al. Infusion therapy standards of practice, 8th edition. J Infus Nurs 2021;44(1S):S1–224.
8. Cies JJ, Moore WS II. Neonatal and peripheral parenteral nutrition: what is a safe osmolarity? Nutr Clin Pract 2014;29(1):118–24.
9. Legemaat M, Carr PJ, van Rens RM, et al. Peripheral intravenous cannulation: complication rates in the neonatal population: a multicenter observational study. J Vasc Access 2016;17(4):360–5.
10. Gomella TL, Eyal FG, Bany-Mohammed F. Venous access: peripheral intravenous catheterization. In: Gomella's neonatology: management, procedures, on-call problems, diseases, and drugs. 8th edition. New York: McGraw-Hill Education; 2020. Available at: https://accesspediatrics.mhmedical.com/book.aspx?bookid=2762#234450642. Accessed on September 12, 2023.
11. Atay S, Sen S, Cukurlu D. Incidence of infiltration/extravasation in newborns using peripheral venous catheter and affecting factors. Rev Esc Enfrerm USP 2018;52: e03360.
12. Kostogloudis MD, Demiri E, Tsimponis A, et al. Severe extravasation injuries in neonates: a report of 34 cases. Pediatr Dermatol 2015;32(6):830–5.

13. Tsunozaki K, Suenaga H, Aoki M, et al. Comparison of dwell time and complications between peripheral venous catheters and midline catheters in infants weighing ≥ 1500 g at birth. Pediatr Int 2023;65(1):e15611.
14. Wilkins CE, Emmerson AJ. Extravasation injuries on regional neonatal units. Arch Dis Child Fetal Neonatal Ed 2004;89(3):F274–5.
15. Murphy T, Bender J, Taub M, et al. The neonatal preventable harm index: a high reliability tool. J Perinatol 2016;36(8):676–80.
16. Nist MD, Harrison TM, Pickler RH, et al. Measures of stress exposure for hospitalized preterm infants. Nurs Res 2020;69(5S Suppl 1):S11–20.
17. Armbruster D, Slaughter J, Stenger M, et al. Neonatal anthropometric measures and peripherally inserted central catheter depth. Adv Neonatal Care 2021;21(4): 314–21.
18. Gomella TL, Eyal FG, Bany-Mohammed F. Venous access: peripherally inserted central catheter. In: Gomella's neonatology: management, procedures, on-call problems, diseases, and drugs. 8th edition. New York: McGraw-Hill Education; 2020. Available at: https://accesspediatrics.mhmedical.com/book.aspx?bookid= 2762#234450642. Accessed on September 12, 2023.
19. Colacchio K, Deng Y, Northrup V, et al. Complications associated with central and non-central venous catheters in a neonatal intensive care unit. J Perinatol 2012; 32(12):941–6.
20. Salonen S, Tammela O, Koivisto AM, et al. Umbilically and peripherally inserted thin central venous catheters have similar risks of complications in very low-birth-weight infants. Clin Pediatr (Phila) 2023;62(11):1361–8.
21. van den Berg J, Lööf Åström J, Olofsson J, et al. Peripherally inserted central catheter in extremely preterm infants: characteristics and influencing factors. J Neonatal Perinatal Med 2017;10(1):63–70.
22. Bashir R, Swarnam K, Vayalthrikkovil S, et al. Association between peripherally inserted central venous catheter insertion site and complication rates in preterm infants. Am J Perinatol 2016;33(10):945–50.
23. Goldwasser B, Baia C, Kim M, et al. Non-central peripherally inserted central catheters in neonatal intensive care: complication rates and longevity of catheters relative to tip position. Pediatr Radiol 2017;47:1676–81.
24. Jain A, Deshpande P, Shah P. Peripherally inserted central catheter tip position and risk of associated complications in neonates. J Perinatol 2013;33(4):307–12.
25. Qin KR, Ensor N, Barnes R, et al. Standard versus long peripheral catheters for multiday IV therapy: a randomized controlled trial. Pediatrics 2021;147(2). e2020000877.
26. Adams DZ, Little A, Vinsant C, et al. The midline catheter: a clinical review. J Emerg Med 2016;51(3):252–8.
27. Leick-Rude MK, Haney B. Midline catheter use in the intensive care nursery. Neonatal Netw 2006;25(3):189–99.
28. Wyckoff MM. Midline catheter use in the premature and full-term infant. J Vasc Access Devices 1999;4(3):26–9.
29. Lesser E, Chhabra R, Brion LP, et al. Use of midline catheters in low birth weight infants. J Perinatol 1996;16(3 Pt 1):205–7.
30. Moran M. Introducing the midline catheter as a new intravenous access device in neonates. Neonatal Intensive Care 1992;5(3):36–42.
31. Swaminathan L, Flanders S, Horowitz J, et al. Safety, and outcomes of midline catheters vs peripherally inserted catheters for patients with short-term indications. A multicenter study. JAMA Intern Med 2022;182(1):50–8.

32. Villalba-Nicolau M, Chover-Sierra E, Saus-Ortega C, et al. Usefulness of midline catheters versus peripheral venous catheters in an inpatient unit: a pilot randomized clinical trial. Nurs Rep 2022;12(4):814–23.
33. Marsh N, Larsen EN, O'Brien C, et al. Safety and efficacy of midline catheters versus peripheral intravenous catheters: a pilot randomized controlled trial. Int J Nurs Pract 2023;29(2):e13110.
34. Qin K, Ensor N, Barnes R, et al. Long peripheral catheters for intravenous access in adults and children: a systematic review of the literature. J Vasc Access 2021; 22(5):767–77.
35. Ring LM, Rana S, Deutsch N. Implementation of a non-sedated procedural pain management practice guideline and order set. Pediatr Nurs 2023;49(1):12–20.
36. Kleidon TM, Schults JA, Wainwright C, et al. Comparison of midline catheters and peripherally inserted central catheters to reduce the need for general anesthesia in children with respiratory disease: a feasibility randomized controlled trial. Paediatr Anaesth 2021;31(9):985–95.
37. Anderson J, Greenwell A, Louderback J, et al. Comparison of outcomes of extended dwell/midline peripheral intravenous catheters and peripherally inserted central catheters in children. J Assoc Vasc Access 2016;21(3):158–64.
38. Östlund Å, Fläring U, Norberg Å, et al. Complications of Pediatric Midline Catheters: A Prospective Observational Pilot Study. Anesth Analg 2022. https://doi.org/10.1213/ANE.0000000000006328.
39. Paterson RS, Chopra V, Brown E, et al. Selection and insertion of vascular access devices in pediatrics: a systematic review. Pediatrics 2020;145(Suppl 3): S243–68.

Mother's Own Milk Versus Donor Human Milk
What's the Difference?

Leslie A. Parker, PhD, APRN*, Rebecca Koernere, PhD, APRN, CPNP-PC,
Keliy Fordham, RN, BSN, Hussah Bubshait, RN, MSN,
Alissandre Eugene, BS, Adrienne Gefre,
Marion Bendixen, PhD, MSN, RN, IBCLC

KEYWORDS

- Donor human milk • Mother's own milk • Human milk • Breast milk
- Premature infant • Neonatal intensive care unit • Nutrition • Very low birth weight

KEY POINTS

- Due to the processing and donor lactation stage, many nutritional, immunologic, and microbial components present in mother's own milk are reduced or eliminated in donor human milk (DHM).
- Protection against prematurity-related complications is reduced when infants are fed high doses of DHM.
- Research is needed to reduce the negative effects of processing and pasteurization on protective components in DHM.

INTRODUCTION

One out of 8 infants in the United States is born preterm, with approximately 16% born at 22 to 32 weeks gestation.[1] Preterm infants are highly susceptible to potentially preventable complications that significantly increase risks of long-term health and neurodevelopmental problems and their associated costs,[2] and which are reduced when infants are fed their own mother's milk (mother's own milk; MOM).[3,4] Research repeatedly shows preterm infants benefit immensely from the consumption of MOM, including decreased risk of short and long-term morbidities, including late-onset sepsis,[4] retinopathy of prematurity (ROP),[5] neurodevelopmental delays,[6,7] bronchopulmonary dysplasia (BPD),[8] feeding intolerance,[9] and necrotizing enterocolitis (NEC).[10,11] MOM also decreases the length of hospitalization as well as the risk of illness and rehospitalization after neonatal intensive care unit (NICU) discharge.[4]

College of Nursing, University of Florida, Box 100187 College of Nursing, Gainesville, FL, USA
* Corresponding author.
E-mail address: Parkela@ufl.edu

Crit Care Nurs Clin N Am 36 (2024) 119–133
https://doi.org/10.1016/j.cnc.2023.09.002
0899-5885/24/© 2023 Elsevier Inc. All rights reserved.
ccnursing.theclinics.com

When MOM is unavailable, the American Academy of Pediatrics, the World Health Organization, and the European Society for Paediatric Gastroenterology Hepatology and Nutrition recommend preterm very low–birth weight (VLBW;<1500 g) infants receive pasteurized donor human milk (DHM).[12,13] Since the publication of these recommendations, the use of DHM in NICUs has risen dramatically, is now considered standard care, and is available in approximately 97% of level 4 NICUs.[14] However, significant nutritional, immunologic, and microbial compositional differences exist between MOM and DHM; thus, DHM may not provide the same protection against complications as MOM.[15] Therefore, the purpose of this review is to summarize the differences between MOM and DHM, the potential effects on health outcomes, and the clinical implications of these differences.

ETIOLOGY OF COMPOSITIONAL DIFFERENCES BETWEEN DONOR HUMAN MILK AND MOTHER'S OWN MILK

Compositional differences between DHM and MOM are generally the result of DHM processing, including Holder pasteurization and multiple freeze-thaw cycles, as well as the lactation stage of donating mothers.

Pasteurization

By far, the most common method to inactivate potentially pathogenic bacteria and viruses in human milk (HM) is Holder pasteurization, where donated milk is heated to 62.5° C for 30 minutes.[16] The Human Milk Banking Association of North America requires that all DHM be tested for the presence of bacteria and not dispensed if it contains more than 1 colony- forming unit of bacteria per microliter.[17] However, Holder pasteurization also reduces and/or eliminates many of the essential nutrients and bioactive components found in MOM, thus potentially reducing its benefits. For example, lysozymes, secretory immunoglobulin A (sIgA), growth factors, lactoferrin, antioxidants, and anti-inflammatory cytokines, which are known to reduce complications related to prematurity, are reduced, or destroyed during pasteurization.[15]

Multiple Freeze-thaw Cycles

DHM is prepared by pooling MOM from approximately 3 to 5 donors and undergoing several freeze-thaw cycles which can damage, decrease, or eliminate important components in MOM.[18] Furthermore, DHM processing involves transferring milk into multiple plastic containers, allowing fat to adhere to the plastic with each transfer.[19]

Lactation Stage of Donors

The vast majority of mothers who donate milk to HM banks are mothers of term-healthy infants between 1 and 6.4 months of age.[18,20] This is important because the lactation stage significantly affects the composition of HM, with milk from mothers of older infants having fewer growth factors, sIgA, lactoferrin, and anti-inflammatory cytokines, which are important for protection against infection and other prematurity-associated complications as well as nutrients essential for adequate growth and development.[21–23]

COMPOSITIONAL DIFFERENCES BETWEEN MOTHER'S OWN MILK AND DONOR HUMAN MILK
Nutritional

Numerous studies have found that DHM contains fewer calories and less nutritional content than MOM.[23] Due to significantly reduced protein, fat, and carbohydrate content, DHM is estimated to average only 17.6 kcal/oz (range: 15.9–20.7 kcal/oz)[18] compared to 23.1 kcal/oz in MOM from mothers of preterm infants.[24] While sufficient protein intake is essential for optimal growth in preterm infants, DHM contains an average of only 1.0 g/dL compared to 2.1 g/dL in preterm MOM.[20,23,24] Furthermore, pasteurization affects the structure of proteins contained in HM, potentially reducing available amino acids for absorption and growth.[25]

Pasteurization and HM processing also reduce the fat content of HM by up to 25%.[20,23] Because fat contributes a high proportion of the total energy content of HM, this may be an important cause of suboptimal growth in infants fed high doses of DHM.[26] In addition, pasteurization completely eliminates bile salt–stimulating lipase. which is abundant in MOM and essential for fat absorption.[27] Finally, carbohydrates are reduced in DHM, further reducing the caloric content.[20,23] See **Table 1** for differences in macronutrient content between DHM and MOM.

Because DHM provides significantly less energy and nutrients, infants fed high doses of DHM are at increased risk for poor growth compared to those fed MOM or formula.[26] These nutritional differences are important because preterm infants are at significant risk of suboptimal growth, which is highly associated with complications and adverse neurocognitive outcomes.[28,29] Infants fed high doses of DHM require careful monitoring to ensure that they are meeting their nutritional needs and growing appropriately. It is possible that HM fortification specific to infants receiving DHM is needed to optimize growth.

Hormones and growth factors, including adipokines, insulin, insulin-like growth factor, and epidermal growth factor, are abundant in MOM but significantly reduced by pasteurization.[30] These elements are abundant in amniotic fluid and facilitate fetal gastrointestinal (GI) maturation and development, preparing the infant for digestion as well as nutrient absorption and metabolism after birth.[31] When infants are born preterm, exposure to these growth-promoting factors abruptly ceases. Because these elements are prevalent in MOM and increased further in preterm MOM, exposure to these elements continues when infants receive MOM. However, feeding infants, DHM, especially during the first days after birth, limits exposure, which may increase the risk of GI complications, impaired digestion, and decreased nutrient absorption.

Micronutrients and trace elements are important for the growth and prevention of complications. Minimal differences in micronutrient content exist between MOM and DHM, including copper, selenium, iodine, iron, magnesium, and bromine.[32] Calcium and phosphorous are also not reduced in DHM,[33] yet levels of alkaline phosphatase are elevated in infants fed high doses of DHM, suggesting an increased risk for osteopenia of prematurity.[34] Sodium plays an important role in infant growth but is significantly decreased in DHM, likely contributing to suboptimal growth in infants fed high doses of DHM.[26,33,35] Sodium supplementation in infants fed DHM has been shown to be safe and to improve growth.[36] Finally, zinc is decreased in DHM, and because of its important role in linear growth, infants receiving high doses of DHM may need additional zinc supplementation.[37]

Table 1 Macronutrient composition of donor human milk and preterm mother's own milk[18,23,33]		
	Donor Human Milk [Mean (Range)]	Preterm Mother's Own Milk (Mean)
Calories (kcal/oz)	17.6 (15.9–20.7)	23.1
Protein (g/dL)	1 (0.8–1.22)	2.1
Fat (g/dL)	3.9 (3.2–4.5)	4.5
Carbohydrates (g/dL)	7.6 (7.3–7.9)	7.5

Nutritional antioxidants, including vitamins C and E, in addition to certain enzymes are abundant in MOM and significantly reduced in DHM.[38] Preterm infants have inherently low antioxidant capacity and are vulnerable to oxidative stress originating from oxygen therapy, mechanical ventilation, parenteral nutrition, and blood transfusions.[39] Thus, exposure to high doses of DHM could potentially increase the risk of oxidative stress, which is associated with morbidities including BPD, ROP, and NEC.[40]

Microbial Differences

MOM contains live bacteria that colonize the infant's intestinal tract.[16,41] The intestinal microbiome is important to infant health, and when dysbiotic (increased pathogenic bacteria or decreased commensal/beneficial bacteria),[42] is associated with adverse outcomes, including NEC and late-onset sepsis.[43] Bacteria present in MOM are generally commensal and differ among individual mothers based on lactation stage, delivery mode, infant sex, maternal body mass index, race, and parity.[41,44] It is therefore likely that each mother's MOM microbiome is unique and personalized to meet their own infant's growth and immunologic needs.[41,44] Whether infants receive DHM or MOM may exert more of an influence on the intestinal microbiome development than other exposures, including the type of HM fortifier (HM or bovine based) and antibiotic exposure.[45,46] Infants who receive DHM have a more similar intestinal microbiome to those fed MOM compared to formula, likely because exposure to formula contributes to significant microbial differences, which may not be beneficial for infants.[47]

Due to pasteurization, DHM is essentially devoid of commensal bacteria, increasing the risk for intestinal inflammation and dysbiosis, which is associated with adverse outcomes including NEC.[45,48] Infants who receive high doses of MOM versus DHM have more of the beneficial intestinal bacteria protective against NEC and have greater microbial diversity, which is associated with improved outcomes.[43,46] MOM may improve several neonatal outcomes in comparison to DHM, including feeding tolerance and growth, which are likely associated with the microbial benefits of MOM colonizing the infant intestinal microbiome.[45,46]

Human milk oligosaccharides (HMOs) are prebiotics that are abundant in HM and aid in the development of a healthy intestinal microbiome. While not reduced as a result of pasteurization due to the lactation stage of donors, the number of HMOs in DHM is less than that in MOM.[49]

Immunologic

MOM contains an abundance of components that protect the infant from infection and support immune development, including immunoglobulins, lactoferrin, cytokines, growth factors, and lysozymes. The concentration of these components is dependent on a variety of factors including lactation stage, gestational age, as well as maternal and infant infection.[21,50–52] DHM does not contain the same quality or quantity of immunologic components as MOM and may be insufficient to meet the needs of preterm infants who are at high risk for infection and have delayed immunologic development. After pasteurization, many anti-infective and immunologic components are significantly reduced and/or eliminated, including immunoglobulins (immunoglobulin [Ig]A, IgM, and IgD), growth factors, lactoferrin, cytokines, and lysozymes (**Table 2**).[21,22,30,49,53]

Immunoglobulins are a key component of MOM and provide passive immunity to the infant, with IgA being the most abundant immunoglobulin and the first line of defense against infection.[30,54] Immunoglobulins originate from the transformation of lymphocytes that migrate from the mother's intestines to her mammary gland and thus contain antibodies directed against microbial antigens in the mother and infant

Table 2	
Effect of pasteurization and processing on bioactive components in donor human milk[21,30,38]	
Component	**Effect of Pasteurization and Processing**
Lactoferrin	Reduced by 44%–91%
sIgA	Reduced by 44%–91%
IgM	Eliminated
IgG	Reduced by 34%
Lysozymes	Reduced by 18%
Anti-inflammatory cytokines	Reduced by 14%–39%
Antioxidants	Reduced by 67%
Microbiota	Eliminated

Abbreviations: IgM, immunoglobulin M; IgG, immunoglobulin G; sIgA, secretory immunoglobulin A.

environments, providing infant-specific protection against infection.[55] IgA levels are decreased by up to 91% in DHM and infant-specific immunologic protection is lacking.[56]

Lactoferrin is an important component of the immune response, which has anti-inflammatory, antimicrobial, and antiviral properties and reduces the risk of NEC.[57] Lactoferrin is significantly reduced by pasteurization and freeze-thaw cycles and is higher in both colostrum and preterm MOM;[53] thus, its level is reduced by up to 91% in DHM.[56]

CLINICAL DIFFERENCES

While extensive research supports the benefits of MOM for infant health, information regarding the benefits of DHM is much more limited. Besides compositional differences due to DHM processing, DHM may provide less protection against complications due to the personalized and dynamic components in MOM, which provide individualized immunomodulatory and nutritional programming during a critical stage of development.

When compared to formula, DHM is associated with a reduced risk of NEC. A 2014 meta-analysis found that DHM reduced the risk of NEC by 2.77-fold in preterm and/or low–birth weight infants.[58] In addition, while a meta-analysis of 4 studies found a 50% risk reduction in the most severe form of NEC (surgical NEC) when DHM was fed compared to formula, it was not statistically significant.[59] Although this research clearly supports the benefits of DHM compared to formula, the evidence is less clear regarding whether DHM provides as much protection against NEC as MOM. While several studies report no difference in risk between infants fed MOM or DHM, infants fed DHM also received some proportion of MOM, and protection may be dependent upon the dose of MOM with limited protection in infants fed exclusively DHM.[26,60]

Other prematurity-related complications are reduced in a dose-dependent manner when infants receive MOM including BPD, ROP, sepsis, feeding intolerance, and developmental delay. However, the protective effects of DHM against these complications are less clear. A 2018 meta-analysis of 18 studies of both randomized controlled trials (RCTs) and observation studies found no difference in BPD when MOM was supplemented with DHM versus formula. However, meta-analyses of the observational studies found that DHM significantly reduced the incidence of BPD.[61] Because RCTs provide the highest level of evidence, additional research is needed to understand the protective nature of DHM more completely. It is important to note that none of the studies directly compared exclusive MOM to exclusive DHM.

Contradictory evidence exists regarding the effect of DHM versus MOM on the incidence of ROP, with some studies indicating no differences, while others finding greater risk reduction, especially of severe ROP when infants receive MOM.[26] Furthermore, while DHM has been shown to reduce feeding intolerance compared to formula, less feeding intolerance has been reported in infants receiving high doses of MOM compared to DHM.[26,46] However, studies used different definitions of feeding intolerance making comparisons between studies difficult. Similar findings exist regarding late-onset sepsis and length of stay with risk reduction seen with the provision of MOM, with significantly less evidence regarding the protective effects of DHM.[4,26,62] Finally, MOM has been associated with improved cognitive outcomes, and this protection may be dose related.[63,64] However, a meta-analysis of 11 studies comparing DHM to formula found insufficient evidence to support the benefits of DHM in neuroprotection[65,] and higher neurodevelopmental scores have been found in infants fed MOM compared to DHM.[34]

Differences between the beneficial effects of MOM compared to DHM are likely multifactorial, including significant differences in the protective components between MOM and DHM as well as the improved growth and nutrition associated with MOM. However, DHM provides protection by eliminating the exposure to formula, which is known to damage the intestinal epithelial border, increase permeability, creates an unhealthy intestinal microbiome, and are associated with an increased inflammatory response, which increases the risk of complications, including NEC.[66] Furthermore, because of limited MOM availability in the first hours and days post-partum, DHM allows an earlier initiation of feedings, which may improve future feeding tolerance.

PERSONALIZATION OF DONOR HUMAN MILK

MOM provides both personalized nutrition and personalized risk-reduction by contributing to the development of the infant's immune system, training of the immune system to stimulate components that regulate the inflammatory response, and building a network of commensal bacteria that help protect against pathogens.[26,67] Yet mothers of preterm infants are at tremendous risk of producing insufficient amounts of MOM to exclusively feed their infants and DHM is often provided in addition to MOM when volume is insufficient to meet the infant's nutritional needs.[68,69]

It may be possible to personalize DHM to be more like MOM by inoculating DHM with MOM.[70–72] Three studies have investigated using DHM as a base in which to place (inoculate) small amounts of either fresh or frozen MOM to personalize the microbial content of DHM. DHM inoculated with amounts as small as 1% or 5% of MOM has a microbial population with similar microbial diversity as MOM after 8 hours. When incubation time is limited to 4 hours, similar microbiota expansion and diversity occur after inoculation with 10% and 30% MOM.[70–72] These findings suggest greater bacterial growth may occur sooner with increasing amounts of MOM transferred to DHM.

It may thus be possible that transferring small amounts of MOM into DHM and incubating over short periods of time may favor a DHM microbial profile similar to MOM, which may lead to influencing personalized infants' gut microbial communities, thus promoting healthier short and long-term outcomes. More research is needed to fully assess the safety and feasibility of this strategy, and the effect on health outcomes prior to implementation in NICUs. However, it is possible that when MOM is not available in sufficient quantities for exclusive MOM feedings, MOM could be proportioned over multiple feedings to support personalized nutrition.

EFFECT ON MOTHER'S OWN MILK CONSUMPTION

Because mothers may be less motivated to pump and provide MOM when DHM is available, several studies have investigated the effect of DHM availability on the consumption of MOM. Studies investigating the overall impact of DHM availability on MOM consumption at NICU discharge have reported no differences or increased rates of MOM consumption, including a 2016 systematic review of 10 studies and a multisite study of 22 NICUs.[73–77]

However, consumption at NICU discharge may not be a true indicator of MOM consumption during the first weeks of life when MOM exposure may provide the greatest protection against complications. Thus, measuring MOM consumption at specific time periods during hospitalization may be important. While several studies report a significant negative effect on MOM consumption during the first weeks after delivery[78–81] following the implementation of a DHM program, others have shown no differences.[82]

Implementation of a DHM program in NICUs is often part of an initiative to increase overall HM consumption, including strategies to facilitate MOM consumption through staff and family awareness of the importance of HM and the promotion of practices that support lactation.[77] It is likely that these strategies facilitate increased lactation success among mothers, thus increasing infant MOM consumption.

ACCEPTANCE BY FAMILIES AND NEONATAL INTENSIVE CARE UNIT STAFF

Information regarding the acceptability of DHM among families and NICU staff is necessary to facilitate increased HM consumption among vulnerable VLBW infants. Although parents in developing countries report concern regarding the safety of DHM, in the United States, DHM is well accepted by parents and NICU staff.[83,84] However, specific attention is needed regarding the acceptability of DHM based on religious beliefs and practices. For example, sharing of HM from unknown mothers is generally prohibited among Muslims who believe consumption of HM creates a milk kinship between the infant and the donating mother as well as between the infant and the donating mother's biological children, thus preventing future marriages.[85] It is important to consider each family individually and respect their cultural and religious practices and beliefs.

To respect parents' autonomy to make well-informed decisions for their infant, it is essential that they are fully aware of the differences between MOM and DHM and the reasons their infant may receive DHM.[86] Many NICUs provide this information immediately after delivery, contained in a bundle combined with general consent for treatment.[87] While early discussions with parents are necessary to facilitate the initiation of HM feedings soon after birth, it may limit comprehension by parents who may be overwhelmed with information and under significant stress.[87] This emphasizes the importance of continued parental support and education throughout the infant's NICU hospitalization to reinforce information regarding DHM, including reasons for use, potential risks and benefits, and its inferiority to MOM. It is critical that parents understand that DHM is not a replacement for MOM but a bridge to initiation of lactation or a supplement when mothers are unable to provide sufficient MOM for exclusive feedings.

Because mothers are often hospitalized for days to weeks prior to preterm delivery, it is possible that conversations regarding DHM and the superiority of MOM could begin antenatally, allowing parents more time to consider, to ask questions, and be fully informed. For parents to receive comprehensive education regarding DHM, it is essential that all staff be educated on the potential risks and benefits of DHM, the differences between MOM and DHM, and provide lactation support to parents to optimize milk production. However, previous research suggests a lack of knowledge regarding the differences between MOM and DHM among NICU staff, leading to inconsistent parental communication, therefore emphasizing the need for standardized counseling regarding DHM.[81]

USE OF DONOR HUMAN MILK IN OTHER POPULATIONS

While DHM is considered standard care for infants born preterm and VLBW, its use in other populations is rapidly increasing.[88] DHM is now used in intensive care units for late preterm and surgical infants, as well as level I nurseries for infants with excessive weight loss and during mother-infant separation, to decrease the potential risk of complications, avoid exposure to formula, and protect exclusive breastfeeding.[89] However, there is limited research in this area, and few studies have found clinical benefits.[90]

Following GI surgery, DHM has not been shown to reduce the incidence of NEC, late-onset sepsis, days needing a central line, or length of hospital stay.[91] However, an exclusive HM diet was associated with less NEC in infants following cardiac surgery.[92] The use of DHM has shown limited clinical benefit for the treatment of hypoglycemia, neonatal abstinence syndrome, or for the protection of exclusive breastfeeding.[90]

IMPLICATIONS FOR RESEARCH

While the use of DHM decreases the risk of NEC in preterm VLBW infants, less evidence exists regarding its protective benefits regarding other complications. Further research is needed to determine whether DHM is associated with a decreased risk of other prematurity-related complications and the extent of this protection. Because it is unethical to randomize infants to be exclusively MOM-fed or DHM-fed, infants in studies regarding the benefits of DHM are generally fed at least some MOM, which may overinflate the extent of protection from DHM. In addition, research is needed to improve DHM by making it more like MOM, including nutritional, microbial, and immunologic composition. Because DHM is considered standard care, it is critical to ensure that DHM is as beneficial as possible.

Research is also needed to elucidate the potential use of DHM in populations other than preterm infants, including whether it improves clinical outcomes and/or protects exclusive breastfeeding. Although parents may prefer their infant be fed DHM instead of formula, DHM is expensive, and while cost-saving in VLBW infants due to a reduction in NEC,[90,93] limited information exists regarding the economic benefits of DHM in other populations. Because DHM is a limited commodity, use in other populations where benefits may be negligible could decrease availability to those most at risk of formula exposure.

Additional research is needed to investigate potential methods besides Holder pasteurization to maintain more of the beneficial components of MOM while continuing to ensure the safety of DHM. Methods including high-temperature short-term pasteurization, high-pressure processing, ultraviolet-C irradiation, and ultrasonication need further research.[53,94]

IMPLICATIONS FOR CLINICAL PRACTICE

Likely, the most important clinical implication regarding the use of DHM is developing and implementing strategies to support mothers to provide MOM, thus reducing the need for DHM. While quality improvement projects have been successful in this endeavor, significant NICU staff commitment is required. In addition, it is essential

Box 1
Summary of clinical significance
Donor human milk (DHM) is recommended when mother's own milk (MOM) is unavailable or volume insufficient to provide exclusive MOM feedings
DHM is inferior to MOM and does not provide the same protection against complications
DHM protects against necrotizing enterocolitis, but this protection is likely diminished compared to MOM
Little is known regarding whether DHM protects against other prematurity-related complications
Infants fed DHM may require additional micronutrient supplementation, including sodium and zinc to promote growth and improve clinical outcomes
Because it contains beneficial bacteria, MOM is critical to normal development of the infant's gastrointestinal microbiome
MOM has increased levels of immunologic components that protect the infant from infection and aid in the development of their immune system
Availability of DHM in neonatal intensive care units (NICUs) does not appear to negatively affect MOM consumption
Parents need information regarding DHM and MOM, which should begin prior to delivery and continue throughout NICU hospitalization
Consideration of families' cultural and religious practices and beliefs concerning DHM is necessary
Research is needed to determine the benefits of DHM in populations other than preterm and very low–birth weight infants, including the risks to exclusive breastfeeding
Mothers should receive ongoing support to facilitate lactation success to increase consumption of MOM

that parents and NICU staff have a clear understanding of the differences between MOM and DHM. Policies and procedures that standardize parental counseling regarding both the risks and benefits of DHM are necessary to assist parents in making informed decisions. Information should emphasize that DHM is not a substitute for MOM but a bridge until MOM is available and/or a supplement when MOM is insufficient to meet the infant's nutritional needs. Education should begin prenatally in high-risk clinics and antenatally prior to delivery, when mothers are not recovering from a potentially difficult delivery.

Additionally, infants who receive high doses of DHM require close monitoring for complications, as well as suboptimal growth. It may be necessary to provide a more individualized HM fortification strategy to promote sufficient growth in these infants. **Box 1** provides an overview of information important for NICU healthcare providers regarding the use of DHM.

SUMMARY

This review of differences between MOM and DHM provides the information necessary for NICU nurses and other health care providers to provide optimal care to infants in the NICU based upon the proportion of DHM versus MOM consumed. Due to HM processing and the lactation stage of donors, many essential nutritional, immunologic, and microbial components are reduced or eliminated in DHM, which decreases protection against complications and may actually increase the risk of poor growth. It is necessary that parents are aware of these differences in order to make informed decisions regarding their infant's care and whether or not they continue providing MOM to their infant. Because MOM is far superior to DHM, it is essential that NICU staff support mothers to continue providing MOM to their infants.

CLINICS CARE POINTS

- Infants receiving high doses of DHM require careful monitoring for complications and poor growth.
- Individualized HM fortification may be needed in infants fed high doses of DHM to optimize growth.
- Parents require information regarding differences between DHM and MOM to make informed decisions.

DISCLOSURE

The authors have nothing to disclose.

REFERENCES

1. March of dimes. (2021). Available at: https://www.marchofdimes.com/peristats/. Accessed August 18, 2023.
2. Anderson JG, Baer RJ, Partridge JC, et al. Survival and major morbidity of extremely preterm infants: a population-based study. Pediatrics 2016;138(1): 2015–4434.
3. Patel A, Engstrom J, Goldman J, et al. Dose response benefits of human milk in extremely low birth weight premature infants. Honolulu, Hawaii: Pediatric Academic Societies; 2008. Presented at.
4. Patel AL, Johnson TJ, Engstrom JL, et al. Impact of early human milk on sepsis and health-care costs in very low birth weight infants. J perinatology 2013;33(7):514–9.
5. Bharwani SK, Green BF, Pezzullo JC, et al. Systematic review and meta-analysis of human milk intake and retinopathy of prematurity: a significant update. J perinatology 2016. https://doi.org/10.1038/jp.2016.98.
6. Vohr BR, Poindexter BB, Dusick AM, et al. Persistent beneficial effects of breast milk ingested in the neonatal intensive care unit on outcomes of extremely low birth weight infants at 30 months of age. Pediatrics 2007;120(4):e953–9.
7. Vohr BR, Poindexter BB, Dusick AM, et al. Beneficial effects of breast milk in the neonatal intensive care unit on the developmental outcome of extremely low birth weight infants at 18 months of age. Pediatrics 2006;118(1):e115–23.
8. Huang J, Zhang L, Tang J, et al. Human milk as a protective factor for bronchopulmonary dysplasia: a systematic review and meta-analysis. Arch Dis Child Fetal Neonatal Ed 2018. https://doi.org/10.1136/archdischild-2017-314205.
9. Assad M, Elliott MJ, Abraham JH. Decreased cost and improved feeding tolerance in VLBW infants fed an exclusive human milk diet. J perinatology 2016; 36(3):216–20.
10. Sullivan S, Schanler RJ, Kim JH, et al. An exclusively human milk-based diet is associated with a lower rate of necrotizing enterocolitis than a diet of human milk and bovine milk-based products. J pediatrics 2010;156(4):562–7.

11. Schanler RJ, Lau C, Hurst NM, et al. Randomized trial of donor human milk versus preterm formula as substitutes for mothers' own milk in the feeding of extremely premature infants. Pediatrics 2005;116(2):400–6.

12. Breastfeeding and the use of human milk. Pediatrics 2012;129(3):e827–41.

13. Meek JY, Noble L. Policy Statement: breastfeeding and the use of human milk. Pediatrics. J 2022;150(1). https://doi.org/10.1542/peds.2022-057988.

14. Boundy EO, Anstey EH, Nelson JM. Donor human milk use in Advanced neonatal care units - United States, 2020. MMWR (Morb Mortal Wkly Rep) 2022;71(33): 1037–41.

15. Peila C, Moro GE, Bertino E, et al. The effect of holder pasteurization on nutrients and biologically-active components in donor human milk: a review. Nutrients 2016;8(8). https://doi.org/10.3390/nu8080477.

16. Abrams SA, Landers S, Noble LM, et al, COMMITTEE ON NUTRITION, SECTION ON BREASTFEEDING, COMMITTEE ON FETUS AND NEWBORN. Donor human milk for the high-risk infant: preparation, safety, and usage options in the United States. Pediatrics 2017;139(1). https://doi.org/10.1542/peds.2016-3440.

17. Clifford V, Klein LD, Sulfaro C, et al. What are optimal bacteriological screening test cut-offs for pasteurized donor human milk intended for feeding preterm infants? J Hum Lactation 2021;37(1):43–51.

18. Young BE, Borman LL, Heinrich R, et al. Effect of pooling practices and time postpartum of milk donations on the energy, macronutrient, and zinc concentrations of resultant donor human milk pools. J pediatrics 2019;214:54–9.

19. Zozaya C, García-Serrano A, Fontecha J, et al. Fat loss in continuous enteral feeding of the preterm infant: How much, what and when is it lost? Nutrients 2018;10(7). https://doi.org/10.3390/nu10070809.

20. Chang FY, Fang LJ, Chang CS, et al. The effect of processing donor milk on its nutrient and energy content. Breastfeed Med 2020;15(9):576–82.

21. Rodríguez-Camejo C, Puyol A, Fazio L, et al. Impact of Holder pasteurization on immunological properties of human breast milk over the first year of lactation. Pediatr Res 2020;87(1):32–41.

22. Lima HK, Wagner-Gillespie M, Perrin MT, et al. Bacteria and bioactivity in Holder pasteurized and shelf-stable human milk products. Curr Dev Nutr 2017;1(8): e001438.

23. Perrin MT, Belfort MB, Hagadorn JI, et al. The Nutritional composition and energy content of donor human milk: a systematic review. Advances nutr 2020;11(4): 960–70.

24. Dietetics PNG. Academy of Nutrition, Guidelines for preparation of human milk in health care facilities. 3rd edition. Chicago, IL: Academy of Nutrition and Dietetics; 2019.

25. Pitino MA, Beggs MR, O'Connor DL, et al. Donor human milk processing and its impact on infant digestion: a systematic scoping review of in vitro and in vivo studies. Adv Nutr 2023;14(1):173–89.

26. Cartagena D, Penny F, McGrath JM, et al. Differences in neonatal outcomes among premature infants exposed to mother's own milk versus donor human milk. (1536-0911 (Electronic)).

27. Baro C, Giribaldi M, Arslanoglu S, et al. Effect of two pasteurization methods on the protein content of human milk. Front Biosci 2011;3(3):818–29.

28. Hickey L, Burnett A, Spittle AJ, et al. Extreme prematurity, growth and neurodevelopment at 8 years: a cohort study. Arch Dis Child 2021;106(2):160–6.

29. Simon L, Théveniaut C, Flamant C, et al. In preterm infants, length growth below expected growth during hospital stay predicts poor neurodevelopment at 2 years. Neonatology 2018;114(2):135–41.

30. Escuder-Vieco D, Espinosa-Martos I, Rodríguez JM, et al. Effect of HTST and Holder pasteurization on the concentration of immunoglobulins, growth factors, and hormones in donor human milk. Front Immunol 2018;9:2222.

31. Wagner CL, Taylor SN, Johnson D. Host factors in amniotic fluid and breast milk that contribute to gut maturation. Clin Rev Allergy Immunol 2008;34(2):191–204.

32. Mohd-Taufek N, Cartwright D, Davies M, et al. The effect of pasteurization on trace elements in donor breast milk. J Perinatol 2016;36(10):897–900.

33. Gates A, Hair AB, Salas AA, et al. Nutrient composition of donor human milk and comparisons to preterm human milk. J Nutr 2023. https://doi.org/10.1016/j.tjnut.2023.07.012.

34. Kazmi SH, Berman S, Caprio M, et al. The impact of donor breast milk on metabolic bone disease, postnatal growth, and neurodevelopmental outcomes at 18 months' corrected age. JPEN (J Parenter Enteral Nutr) 2022;46(3):600–7.

35. Perrin MT, Friend LL, Sisk PM. Fortified donor human milk frequently does not meet sodium recommendations for the preterm infant. J Pediatr 2022;244:219–23.

36. Isemann B, Mueller EW, Narendran V, et al. Impact of early sodium supplementation on hyponatremia and growth in premature infants: a randomized controlled trial. JPEN (J Parenter Enteral Nutr) 2016;40(3):342–9.

37. Staub E, Evers K, Askie LM. Enteral zinc supplementation for prevention of morbidity and mortality in preterm neonates. Cochrane Database Syst Rev 2021; 3(3):Cd012797.

38. Hanson C, Lyden E, Furtado J, et al. A comparison of nutritional antioxidant content in breast milk, donor milk, and infant formulas. Nutrients 2016;8(11). https://doi.org/10.3390/nu8110681.

39. Sandal G, Uras N, Gokmen T, et al. Assessment of oxidant/antioxidant system in newborns and their breast milks. J maternal-fetal & neo medicine 2013;26(5):540–3.

40. de Almeida VO, Pereira RA, Amantéa SL, et al. Neonatal diseases and oxidative stress in premature infants: an integrative review. J Pediatr 2022;98(5):455–62. https://doi.org/10.1016/j.jped.2021.11.008.

41. Moossavi S, Sepehri S, Robertson B, et al. Composition and variation of the human milk microbiota are influenced by maternal and early-life factors. Cell Host Microbe 2019;25(2):324–35.e4.

42. Petersen C, Round JL. Defining dysbiosis and its influence on host immunity and disease. Cell Microbiol 2014;16(7):1024–33.

43. Pammi M, Cope J, Tarr PI, et al. Intestinal dysbiosis in preterm infants preceding necrotizing enterocolitis: a systematic review and meta-analysis. Microbiome 2017;5(1):31.

44. Lyons KE, Shea CO, Grimaud G, et al. The human milk microbiome aligns with lactation stage and not birth mode. Sci Rep 2022;12(1):5598.

45. Kumbhare SV, Jones WD, Fast S, et al. Source of human milk (mother or donor) is more important than fortifier type (human or bovine) in shaping the preterm infant microbiome. Cell Rep Med 2022;3(9):100712.

46. Ford SL, Lohmann P, Preidis GA, et al. Improved feeding tolerance and growth are linked to increased gut microbial community diversity in very-low-birth-weight infants fed mother's own milk compared with donor breast milk. Am J Clin Nutr 2019;109(4):1088–97.

47. Parra-Llorca A, Gormaz M, Alcántara C, et al. Preterm gut microbiome depending on feeding type: significance of donor human milk. Front Microbiol 2018;9:1376.
48. Cong X, Judge M, Xu W, et al. Influence of feeding type on gut microbiome development in hospitalized preterm infants. Nurs Res 2017;66(2):123–33.
49. Marx C, Bridge R, Wolf AK, et al. Human milk oligosaccharide composition differs between donor milk and mother's own milk in the NICU. J Hum Lactation 2014; 30(1):54–61.
50. Turin CG, Zea-Vera A, Rueda MS, et al. Lactoferrin concentration in breast milk of mothers of low-birth-weight newborns. J Perinatol 2017;37(5):507–12.
51. Breakey AA, Hinde K, Valeggia CR, et al. Illness in breastfeeding infants relates to concentration of lactoferrin and secretory Immunoglobulin A in mother's milk. Evol Med Public Health 2015;2015(1):21–31.
52. Trend S, Strunk T, Lloyd ML, et al. Levels of innate immune factors in preterm and term mothers' breast milk during the 1st month postpartum. Br J Nutr 2016; 115(7):1178–93.
53. Dussault N, Cayer MP, Landry P, et al. Comparison of the effect of Holder pasteurization and high-pressure processing on human milk bacterial load and bioactive factors preservation. J Pediatr Gastroenterol Nutr 2021;72(5):756–62.
54. Czosnykowska-Łukacka M, Lis-Kuberka J, Królak-Olejnik B, et al. Changes in human milk immunoglobulin profile during prolonged lactation. Front Pediatr 2020; 8:428.
55. Zhu J, Dingess KA, Mank M, et al. Personalized profiling reveals donor- and lactation-specific trends in the human milk proteome and peptidome. J Nutr 2021;151(4):826–39.
56. Arroyo G, Ortiz Barrientos KA, Lange K, et al. Effect of the various steps in the processing of human milk in the concentrations of IgA, IgM, and cactoferrin. Breastfeeding med 2017;12(7):443–5.
57. Kell DB, Heyden EL, Pretorius E. The biology of lactoferrin, an iron-binding protein that can help defend against viruses and bacteria. Front Immunol 2020;11: 1221.
58. Quigley M, McGuire W. Formula versus donor breast milk for feeding preterm or low birth weight infants. Cochrane Database Syst Rev 2014;4:CD002971.
59. Silano M, Milani GP, Fattore G, et al. Donor human milk and risk of surgical necrotizing enterocolitis: a meta-analysis. Clin Nutr 2019;38(3):1061–6.
60. Altobelli E, Angeletti PM, Verrotti A, et al. The impact of human milk on necrotizing enterocolitis: a systematic review and meta-analysis. Nutrients 2020;12(5). https://doi.org/10.3390/nu12051322.
61. Villamor-Martínez E, Pierro M, Cavallaro G, et al. Donor human milk protects against bronchopulmonary dysplasia: a systematic review and meta-analysis. Nutrients 2018;10(2). https://doi.org/10.3390/nu10020238.
62. Cortez J, Makker K, Kraemer DF, et al. Maternal milk feedings reduce sepsis, necrotizing enterocolitis and improve outcomes of premature infants. J Perinatol 2018; 38(1):71–4.
63. Horta BL, Loret de Mola C, Victora CG. Breastfeeding and intelligence: a systematic review and meta-analysis. Acta Paediatr 2015;104(467):14–9.
64. Victora CG, Horta BL, Loret de Mola C, et al. Association between breastfeeding and intelligence, educational attainment, and income at 30 years of age: a prospective birth cohort study from Brazil. Lancet Global Health 2015;3(4):e199–205.
65. Quigley M, Embleton ND, McGuire W. Formula versus donor breast milk for feeding preterm or low birth weight infants. Cochrane Database Syst Rev 2018; 6(6):Cd002971.

66. Aguilar-Lopez M, Wetzel C, MacDonald A, et al. Metagenomic profile of the fecal microbiome of preterm infants consuming mother's own milk with bovine milk-based fortifier or infant formula: a cross-sectional study. Am J Clin Nutr 2022; 116(2):435–45.

67. Nash MJ, Frank DN, Friedman JE. Early microbes modify immune system development and metabolic homeostasis-the "restaurant" hypothesis revisited. Front Endocrinol 2017;8:349.

68. Bendixen MM, Weaver MT, Parker LA. Milk volume outcomes in pump-dependent mothers of critically Ill infants. Adv Neonatal Care 2022;22(3).

69. Murase M, Nommsen-Rivers L, Morrow AL, et al. Predictors of low milk volume among mothers who delivered preterm. J Hum Lact 2014;30(4):425–35.

70. Cacho NT, Harrison NA, Parker LA, et al. Personalization of the microbiota of donor human milk with mother's own milk. Front Microbiol 2017;8:1470.

71. Torrez Lamberti MF, Harrison NA, Bendixen MM, et al. Frozen Mother's Own Milk Can Be Used Effectively to Personalize Donor Human Milk. (1664-302X (Print)).

72. Mallardi D, Tabasso C, Piemontese P, et al. Inoculation of mother's own milk could personalize pasteurized donor human milk used for feeding preterm infants. J Transl Med 2021;19(1):420.

73. Tshamala D, Pelecanos A, Davies MW. Factors associated with infants receiving their mother's own breast milk on discharge from hospital in a unit where pasteurised donor human milk is available. J Paediatr Child Health 2018. https://doi.org/10.1111/jpc.14062.

74. Parker MG, Barrero-Castillero A, Corwin BK, et al. Pasteurized human donor milk use among US level 3 neonatal intensive care units. J Hum Lactation 2013;29(3): 381–9.

75. Williams T, Nair H, Simpson J, et al. Use of donor human milk and maternal breastfeeding rates: a systematic review. J Hum Lactation 2016;32(2):212–20.

76. Kantorowska A, Wei JC, Cohen RS, et al. Impact of donor milk availability on breast milk use and necrotizing enterocolitis rates. Pediatrics 2016;137(3): e20153123.

77. Corallo J, Bieda A, Garland M, et al. The impact of a donor human milk program on the provision of mothers' own milk at discharge in very low birth weight infants. J Perinatol 2022;42(11):1473–9.

78. Esquerra-Zwiers A, Wicks J, Rogers L. Impact of donor human milk in a high mother's own milk feeding neonatal intensive care unit presented at: 17th International Society for Research in Human Milk and Lactation. South Carolina: Kiawah Island; 2017.

79. Utrera Torres MI, Medina Lopez C, Vazquez Roman S, et al. Does opening a milk bank in a neonatal unit change infant feeding practices? A before and after study. Int Breastfeed J 2010;5:4.

80. Delfosse NM, Ward L, Lagomarcino AJ, et al. Donor human milk largely replaces formula-feeding of preterm infants in two urban hospitals. J Perinatol 2013;33(6): 446–51.

81. Parker LA, Cacho N, Engelmann C, et al. Consumption of mother's own milk by infants born extremely preterm following implementation of a donor human milk program: a retrospective cohort study. J Pediatr 2019;211:33–8.

82. Marinelli KA, Lussier MM, Brownell E, et al. The effect of a donor milk policy on the diet of very low birth weight infants. J Hum Lactation 2014;30(3):310–6.

83. Jahan Y, Rahman S, Shamsi T, et al. Attitudes and views concerning human milk banking among mothers residing in a rural region of Bangladesh. J Human Lactation 2022;38(1):108–17.

84. Magowan S, Burgoine K, Ogara C, et al. Exploring the barriers and facilitators to the acceptability of donor human milk in eastern Uganda - a qualitative study. Int Breastfeed J 2020;15(1):28.
85. Subudhi S, Sriraman N. Islamic beliefs about milk kinship and donor human milk in the United States. Pediatrics 2021;147(2). https://doi.org/10.1542/peds.2020-0441.
86. McGlothen-Bell K, Cleveland L, Pados BF. To consent, or not to consent, that is the question: ethical issues of informed consent for the use of donor human milk in the NICU Setting. Adv Neonatal Care 2019;19(5):371–5.
87. Esquerra-Zwiers A, Rossman B, Meier P, et al. "It's somebody else's milk": unraveling the tension in mothers of preterm infants who provide consent for pasteurized donor human milk. J human lactation 2016;32(1):95–102.
88. Belfort MB, Drouin K, Riley JF, et al. Prevalence and trends in donor milk use in the well-baby nursery: a survey of northeast United States birth hospitals. Breastfeed Med 2018;13(1):34–41.
89. Lewis SC, McMahon M, Combs G, et al. The nuts and bolts of implementing a pasteurized donor human milk program on a mother baby unit. J human lactation 2018;34(1):116–9.
90. McCune S, Perrin MT. Donor human milk use in populations other than the preterm infant: a systematic scoping review. Breastfeed Med 2021;16(1):8–20.
91. Hoban R, Khatri S, Patel A, et al. Supplementation of mother's own milk with donor milk in infants with gastroschisis or intestinal atresia: a retrospective study. Nutrients 2020;12(2). https://doi.org/10.3390/nu12020589.
92. Cognata A, Kataria-Hale J, Griffiths P, et al. Human milk use in the preoperative period is associated with a lower risk for necrotizing enterocolitis in neonates with complex congenital heart disease. J Pediatr 2019;215:11–6.e2.
93. Zanganeh M, Jordan M, Mistry H. A systematic review of economic evaluations for donor human milk versus standard feeding in infants. Matern Child Nutr 2021;17(2):e13151.
94. Moro GE, Billeaud C, Rachel B, et al. Processing of donor human milk: update and recommendations from the European Milk Bank Association (EMBA). Front Pediatr 2019;7:49.

Perspectives on Telehealth Use with the Neonatal Population

Policy, Practice, and Implementation Considerations

Danielle Altares Sarik, PhD, APRN, CPNP-PC[a],*,
Yui Matsuda, PhD, PHNA-BC, MPH[b], Kelli Garber, DNP, APRN, PPCNP-BC[c],
Melody Hernandez, MD, PhD, RN[a],
Evelyn Abrahante Terrell, OTD, MHSA[a]

KEYWORDS

- Neonatal • NICU • Telehealth • Transition of care • Hospital to home

KEY POINTS

- Telehealth has proven to be a valuable tool in managing the neonatal and pediatric population, including high-risk children with medical complexity.
- Telehealth can be used to help support the transition from hospital to home, provide remote monitoring to neonates, and extend the reach of pediatric subspecialists with neonatal expertise to underserved and rural communities.
- Clinicians are responsible to understand laws and regulations that govern telehealth practice.
- While using telehealth, clinicians should strive for an equity-focused approach to ensure all families can receive high-quality, culturally appropriate care.

INTRODUCTION

Telehealth, also referred to as telemedicine, is an innovative technology that has seen a surge in use during the last several years. Defined as the use of electronic information and telecommunications technologies to support and promote long-distance clinical health care, patient and professional health-related education, and public health

[a] Nicklaus Children's Hospital, 3100 SW 62nd Avenue, Miami, FL 33155, USA; [b] University of Miami School of Nursing and Health Studies, 5030 Brunson Drive, Coral Gables, FL 33146, USA; [c] Old Dominion University School of Nursing, Virginia Beach Center, 1881 University Drive, Virginia Beach, VA 23453, USA
* Corresponding author. 3100 SW 62nd Avenue, Miami, FL 33155.
E-mail address: Danielle.sarik@nicklaushealth.org

Crit Care Nurs Clin N Am 36 (2024) 135–146
https://doi.org/10.1016/j.cnc.2023.09.003
0899-5885/24/© 2023 Elsevier Inc. All rights reserved.

and health administration,[1] the growing popularity of this modality ensures that most providers and patients in the United States have either personally used or engaged in care through telehealth.[2,3] Telehealth can provide tangible benefits for the pediatric population and children with medical complexity, including decreasing emergency room use or hospital readmission[4] and preventing potential exposure to communicable diseases. For the neonatal population, telehealth can offer benefits across the care continuum through increased access to care,[5] early intervention, increased convenience, reduced costs,[6] and improved continuity of care,[7] all of which may have a positive effect on quality outcomes.[4,8–10] Moreover, telehealth care models may address social determinants of health (SDOH), increase equity, and reduce disparities by extending the reach of providers to underserved communities.[11]

The purpose of this article is to review the policy and practice implications of telehealth use with the neonatal population. The authors provide a brief history of neonatal care, discuss how telehealth has been used in the neonatal population, provide an overview of policy and legislative considerations, and discuss how to continue telehealth expansion.

Care of the Neonatal Population: History and Potential Use of Telehealth

As a pediatric subspecialty, neonatology began to gain recognition and attention in the 1960s.[12] Owing to the advancements in neonatology and neonatal nursing, the health outcomes of neonates and infants have significantly improved. For example, although infants with a birth weight of 1 kg in the 1960s had a 95% mortality risk, by the 2000s, the probability of survival increased to 95%.[12] In addition, the edge of viability, a term that refers to the age at which a premature infant can survive with medical intervention, continues to fall.[13] Today, almost one in every 10 newborns in the United States receives care in the neonatal intensive care unit (NICU) within their first month of life, and admission rates continue to increase.[14]

When providing care to a neonate, especially in intensive care settings such as the NICU, it is important to recognize the interconnected nature of the patient and caregiver. Referred to as dyad care, interventions that promote the bond between the caregiver and infant may include skin-to-skin holding, performing evaluations and treatment within close proximity to the caregiver, and ensuring support for the caregiver to provide optimal care for the infant. The family-centered care model views caregivers as integral team members in a neonate's care,[15] ensuring that caregivers are present and active participants in the hands-on experience with their infant, which helps to facilitate caregivers' confidence and knowledge regarding infant care.

After discharge, caregivers of infants in the NICU encounter multiple transitions of care, starting from the delivery team and neonatologists to their community pediatricians and specialists, in addition to assuming primary responsibility for their infant. Common challenges faced by under-resourced caregivers and families with infants include the potential loss of medical coverage, lack of access to medical professionals, and social and economic issues, resulting in health disparities.[5] Although caregivers may face multiple challenges with the transition of care, telehealth is a powerful tool to continue supporting dyad care during this critical period.

EXAMPLES OF TELEHEALTH USE AMONG THE NEONATAL POPULATION
Telehealth Subspecialty Consultation Services for Community Neonatal Intensive Care Units

Large pediatric medical centers and specialty hospitals are in a position to connect pediatric subspecialists with neonatal expertise in underserved communities. Cross-sector collaborations bring systems together, helps address workforce challenges, and transforms care for rural and underserved communities. One example of such collaboration exists at Nicklaus Children's Hospital (Nicklaus). Through a expanded partnership with affiliate health systems in South Florida, Nicklaus became a regional resource through a NICU telehealth consultation program launched in May 2023. The telehealth model and workflows provide access to more than 70 pediatric specialists in 12 subspecialties, facilitating virtual inpatient visits, peer-to-peer consultations, and streamlining facility transfers for neonates with high acuity requiring a higher level of care. The success of this partnership demonstrates that community collaborative alliances using telehealth have the ability to break down geographic barriers to subspecialty neonatal care.

Virtual Transition of Care Support from the Neonatal Intensive Care Units to the Community

While hospitalized, patients and families benefit from the support and guidance of the clinical care team, including nurses, physicians, social workers, and pharmacists. However, at the point of discharge from the hospital, care is transitioned from the inpatient care team to the family or caregiver and outpatient providers. This period of acute transition represents a time of increased stress and may also pose additional risks for medical reutilization, such as readmission or use of an emergency room or an urgent care center.[16] During the acute transition period, infants and families may not have immediate access to outpatient specialty providers and may experience gaps in health care access.

The Baby Steps model, a nurse-led telehealth transition of care intervention, was developed to address this gap.[4] The model uses telehealth, provided by a trained neonatal registered nurse (RN), as a way to ease the transition into the community for infants and caregivers, as well as bridge the gap in access that many families and caregivers, those with financial hardships, experience. After discharge, caregivers are contacted via telehealth within 48 to 72 hours, and the infant and caregiver are assessed for any nursing or psychosocial needs. Anticipatory guidance, medication support, and nursing care are reviewed with caregivers, and referrals to higher levels of care are made as needed. In the first 3 years of this program, close to 700 patients and families have received support through Baby Steps, and the program has demonstrated significant reductions in 30-day readmission, 30-day emergency room or urgent care use, and high levels of caregiver satisfaction.[5]

DISCUSSION
Policy and Legislative Considerations for Telehealth Use with the Neonatal Population

RNs and advanced practice RNs (APRNs) interested in using telehealth in their practice must be well-versed in matters of health policy. The RN and APRN are responsible for being familiar with the laws and regulations that govern their practice, and telehealth care is no different. Telehealth policy is constantly evolving, particularly because the COVID-19 pandemic and related public health emergency (PHE) was declared and later rescinded.[17] Legislation and regulation at both the federal and state levels impact telehealth care delivery, necessitating an understanding of both telehealth-specific and broader health care statutes, rules, and regulations.[18] Telehealth-related policy determines who can deliver telemedicine services and to whom, in what location, via which modality, and whether it will be reimbursed.[19]

Federal-level policy considerations

Pandemic-related changes to telehealth policy. During the COVID-19 PHE, many policies considered barriers to telehealth adoption were relaxed to expand access to care via telecommunication tools and technologies.[20] At the federal level, these included changes to Medicare, such as the removal of geographic restrictions on originating sites, expanded provider types at distant sites, allowing the home as an originating site, and the allowance of audio-only communication platforms.[20] In addition, exceptions were granted regarding prescribing controlled substances via telehealth. The Ryan Haight Act of 2008 requires that an in-person visit is completed before prescribing controlled substances via telehealth unless the patient is in a facility or in the physical presence of a provider who holds a Drug Enforcement Administration (DEA) registration. During the PHE, this in-person examination requirement was removed and provided specific expectations were met.[21,22] Before the PHE, providers were required to hold a DEA registration in each state where controlled substances were prescribed. This requirement was also waived during the PHE.[22] Some of these telehealth flexibilities have been made permanent, whereas others remain temporary,[1,22] with various bills having been introduced to ensure their permanence.

Reimbursement. Following the end of the COVID-19 PHE, the Centers for Medicare & Medicaid Services continue to provide coverage for telehealth services delivered by physicians and other eligible professionals to Medicare beneficiaries in the home setting. Recent legislation enabled an extension of many of the Medicare telehealth flexibilities and waivers implemented during the PHE through December 31, 2024. Clinicians bill for telehealth services under the Medicare Physician Fee Schedule in the same way as during the PHE. Congressional action is essential for sustainability and continued advancement of telehealth innovation beyond December 2024, when current waivers enacted by Congress will expire.[18]

State-level considerations

Expanded access. At the state level, similar modifications were made during the PHE by Medicaid programs, expanding access to care for many families. In addition to Medicaid policies that govern telehealth care, many states now have specific telehealth laws or telemedicine acts. These statutes may be significantly different between states. State telehealth laws often include a definition of telehealth or telemedicine, guidelines pertaining to establishing a patient–provider relationship via telehealth, prescribing information, practice standards, consent requirements, out-of-state provider requirements, and certification requirements.[20] When reviewing state telehealth laws, individuals and health systems must evaluate what legislation they modify if they are stand-alone and whether the language extends to RN and/or APRN practice.[17] In addition, it is important for nurses to review their state's Nurse Practice Act and any advisory opinions or position statements published by licensing boards regarding telehealth nursing practice, as these also vary significantly by state.[23]

Reimbursement. The healthcare industry is bullish on the growing use of telehealth, and many major payers continue to support equitable payment for telehealth services.[24] A state Medicaid policy review for the period of January and March 2023 demonstrated that in 50 states and Washington, DC, reimbursement was available for certain live video encounters.[25] States with payment parity policies have been shown to have higher telehealth utilization. Supporting state-level payment policies will ensure the long-term viability of virtual care.[26]

Licensure. One very important state-level consideration is that of licensure. The patient's physical location is considered the site of service and therefore requires the nurse or provider to be licensed in that state.[27] RNs and APRNs must verify the patient's location at the time services are rendered to ensure they are compliant. If the patient population to be served extends beyond the nurse's primary licensure state, plans should be developed to ensure appropriate licensing before services begin. One solution is a multistate license. The Nurse Licensure Compact (NLC) allows RNs to practice across state lines to any of the 41 compact states in person or via telehealth without requiring an additional license.[28] Depending on the state, a multistate license must be requested rather than automatically granted, so it is important for RNs to research their individual state's procedures and requirements.[28] The NLC does not apply to APRNs. The APRN Compact has yet to be implemented as at least seven states must enact the legislation before it takes effect, and only three have done so as of this writing (Delaware, North Dakota, and Utah).[29]

Position statements and nursing telehealth practice

Familiarity with position statements and guidelines pertaining to nursing specialties and roles from professional organizations is also necessary for clinicians engaging in telehealth use with neonatal populations. Although there is currently no specific position statement about telehealth and neonatal nursing, the American Association of Nurse Practitioners (AANPs) and the American Nurses Association support virtual care while affirming that these services are not a separate specialty or type of care and do not alter the standards of care and professional practice expected with in-person care.[30,31] The AANP also supports the regulation and reimbursement of services on par with the same services delivered in person.[25] In addition, attention should be directed at establishing and demonstrating competencies for the care to be provided via telehealth. This will ensure safe, effective, high-quality care is provided with a patient and family-centered team-based approach.[25]

Advocacy for telehealth

Healthcare organizations and clinicians, together with policymakers, payers, and community leaders, must advocate for telehealth and continue educating patients and families on the value of this modality. Clinicians should support cross-sector collaborations and develop shared priorities using a multipronged approach that includes legislative, regulatory, and state-based advocacy efforts. Organizations may support or endorse legislation to assist patients or clients in sustaining telehealth services and Omni-channel care models, including in-person and virtual care. Advocacy efforts may focus on specific priorities, including

- Advancing permanent telehealth reform that expands the scope of clinicians eligible to provide telehealth services, does not restrict provider type, and ensures access to clinicians, including APRNs, physician assistants, therapists, and RNs.
- Removing restrictions related to patient location necessary to receive telehealth
- Supporting legislation to allow a patient's home to serve as the originating site for telehealth
- Supporting licensure compacts, portability, and telehealth authorization by state licensing boards to facilitate telehealth across state borders
- Supporting continued telehealth coverage and equitable reimbursement by Medicaid and commercial insurers[18,32]

PROTECTING NEONATAL PATIENT AND FAMILY PRIVACY
Health Insurance Portability and Accountability Act Considerations for Clinicians Using Telehealth

The key to telehealth nursing practice is an understanding of the Health Insurance Portability and Accountability Act (HIPAA) of 1996 and its implications for telehealth. HIPAA is a federal law implemented to protect patient health information (PHI) from being disclosed without the patient's consent or knowledge.[33] The HIPAA Privacy Rule addresses the use and disclosure of individuals' health information, whereas the HIPAA Security Rule safeguards PHI that is created, received, maintained, or transmitted electronically.[28] All telehealth care provided by covered entities must comply with the HIPAA rules. Technology that is HIPAA-compliant and secure should always be used. Health care organizations should select technology vendors that agree to follow HIPAA rules and then enter into a business associate agreement pertaining to the telecommunication technologies they are providing.[34] In addition, nurses should ensure that care provided via telehealth is conducted in a private location using headphones to ensure patient privacy.

Telehealth and Social Determinants of Health and Equity-focused Care Approach

When considering the use of telehealth to support the care of the neonatal population, telehealth care providers and supporting team members should strive for an equity-focused approach. Equity in health is defined as the state in which everyone has a fair opportunity to attain their highest level of health,[35] and telehealth is a powerful modality to provide equity-focused care. Nurses' keen assessment can assist with addressing SDOH during the critical transition period from NICU to home. In particular, telehealth care providers need to be aware that the lack of access to technology may inhibit infants and their caregivers from receiving telehealth care at all, or culturally inappropriate care and language discordance may discourage caregivers from seeking telehealth care.

Understanding SDOH is critical for any clinician promoting an equity-focused approach in telehealth among the neonatal population. SDOH are defined as the conditions in the environments where people are born, live, learn, work, play, worship, and age that affects a wide range of health, functioning, and quality-of-life outcomes and risks.[36] Thus, understanding families' home environment and their life context is essential to providing high-quality telehealth care. Connecting within the community setting provides opportunities for nurses to assess the clinical status of infants and their caregivers and their physical, psychological, social, and spiritual environment. Such assessment could then lead to appropriate referral to community providers, organizations, and resources.

Two important aspects need to be considered when engaging in the equity-focused provision of telehealth care: (1) technology access and (2) culturally appropriate and language-concordant care.

Telehealth Access and the Digital Divide

Electronic device access

Access to an appropriate electronic device is a prerequisite to receiving care via telehealth. According to the Pew Research Center, at least 95% of the US population between the ages of 18 and 49 years, which the majority of the caregivers of infants fall into, own a smartphone.[37] However, some families may not have broadband Internet services and have limited data plans, which limit their access to telehealth services.[38] Thus, if a caregiver lacks the financial resources to maintain consistent smartphone and Internet service, disparities in access may occur. Programs, such as the Federal

Communications Commission Wireless and Affordable Connectivity Program,[39] attempt to address this barrier by offering qualified Medicaid recipients and other eligible low-income families the opportunity to receive benefits, including a free smartphone with a discounted plan, facilitating access to health care services.

Digital literacy

Digital literacy, defined as an individual's ability to search and evaluate information on various digital platforms,[40] plays a role in whether caregivers feel able to use a telehealth care platform. Orientation to telehealth applications and test calls before discharge from the clinical setting represents one strategy to mitigate digital literacy challenges.

Ease of access to telehealth platforms

Ease of access to and use of the telehealth platform is also critical.[41] The telehealth platform instructions and questions should be available in multiple languages, aligning with those most commonly used by patients in the geographic catchment of the clinical setting. One strategy to reduce connectivity challenges associated with application use is to minimize the number of steps required to join a virtual visit. Platform features may involve a simplified or single sign-in and support integration with the electronic health record to streamline workflows (e.g., registration process, scheduling virtual appointments). Appointment reminders may be sent through SMS text and email calendar invitations to help avoid missed visits. An additional strategy is to offer various channels to schedule appointments, including scheduling hotlines, online patient portals, and flexibility in scheduling appointments, both before discharge and at visit checkout.

Cultural Appropriateness and Language Concordance

An additional aspect to consider in the equity-focused provision of telehealth care is providing culturally appropriate and language-concordant services. Culturally and Linguistically Appropriate Services (CLAS) Standards clearly articulate our obligation to provide such care and patients' rights to receive such care by law.[42] However, healthcare providers may not be aware of their obligations, and patients may not be aware of their rights. Telehealth providers need to be educated about their responsibilities and patients' rights and ensure that they advocate for their neonatal patients and their caregivers.

Providing culturally appropriate care, defined as a set of behaviors and attitudes that enable effective work in cross-cultural settings, is critical.[43] The concept of culturally appropriate care has been widely discussed in health care; however, as patients come from diverse cultural backgrounds, telehealth providers need to adapt to such diversities. Concepts, such as cultural humility, or the ability to maintain other-oriented stances in regard to patients'/families' cultural identity important to each person, can help to guide the telehealth provider during virtual encounters.[44] Cultural humility emphasizes life-long reflection and acknowledgment of the power imbalance between patients/families and health care providers.[45] Another concept to apply is cultural safety, which is focused on health care providers and patients/families learning together by sharing respect, meaning, knowledge, and experience to create spiritually, socially, emotionally, and physically safe environments.[46] Telehealth care providers are challenged to be reflective in their practice and to create an environment where infants and caregivers feel safe.[17,44,46] In regard to providing language-concordant services, there are several ways to provide such care. One option is the use of a virtual interpreter service, which allows interpreters to join by video to address language barriers. Alternatively, if medical interpreters are available inperson at a health care setting, a telehealth care provider and a medical interpreter can be in the same physical room to provide language-concordant services. Telehealth providers should be trained and competent in collaborating with medical interpreters, regardless of the method.

IMPLEMENTATION CONSIDERATIONS
Education and Competencies

In order to have a cadre of neonatal providers who can effectively administer care through telehealth, robust training is critical. Simulation is a technique that realistically imitates scenarios so that learners can experience telehealth delivery, coupled with guidance and reflection.[47] One such approach, the Baby Steps Telehealth Nursing Simulation program, was developed for undergraduate nursing students so that these students have an opportunity to develop telehealth nursing competencies. The program has allowed nursing students to experience telehealth visits with infants and their caregivers so that students learn how to assess the infant, the caregiver, their interactions, and the home environment in a virtual setting.[48]

In addition to education at the university level, training and competencies must be delivered and evaluated in the health care setting for any provider engaging in telehealth with neonatal populations. Such training can help educate on best practices for telehealth, ensure compliance with state and federal laws and regulations, and promote approaches that consider SDOH and health equity issues.

Reimbursement

Historically, legislation has excluded RNs from professionals eligible to deliver reimbursable telehealth services. This is challenging for the growth and sustainability of innovative nurse-led telehealth service delivery models in primary care practice, disease management, care coordination, and transition of care. In contrast, other members of the health care team, including physicians and APRNs, are able to provide similar services and receive reimbursement. Future legislation and alternative payment models would need to consider RNs as the key members of the health care team permitted to deliver reimbursable telehealth services.[49]

Evaluation

An essential component of a neonatal telehealth program is evaluation. Various frameworks to evaluate the impact of telehealth on the care delivered exist, including the National Quality Forum framework,[50] the World Health Organization framework,[51] and the Agency for Health Research and Quality technical brief.[52] Building off this foundation, Supporting Pediatric Research on Outcomes and Utilization of Telehealth (SPROUT), a part of the American Academy of Pediatrics Section on Telehealth Care, developed the SPROUT Telehealth Evaluation and Measurement profile, which combines these concepts into a single framework to study telehealth's impact on patients.[53] This framework includes four domains: health outcomes, health delivery (quality and cost), patient and provider experience, and program implementation key performance indicators. Findings from the telehealth program evaluation focused on these key areas can facilitate data-driven reimbursement and policy changes. The goal is to communicate telehealth's value to key stakeholders: patients, providers, health systems, and payers.[53] Understanding these factors may facilitate RNs and APRNs to contribute to the continuous quality improvement of telehealth initiatives.

SUMMARY

The use of telehealth with the neonatal population holds great promise. However, in order to use this modality to the fullest, providers need to be aware of and address multiple issues, including federal and state laws and regulations, health equity considerations, and how to manage SDOH that may impact access to services. Multiple programs using telehealth serve as exemplars of how this technology can be leveraged to support the care of neonates and their families.

CLINICS CARE POINTS

- When caring for neonates and their caregivers using telehealth, providers should use a family-centered care approach to optimally care for the dyad.
- It is the responsibility of the registered nurse (RN) and advanced practice RN (APRN) to be familiar with the laws and regulations that govern telehealth practice:
  - State telehealth laws often include a definition of telehealth or telemedicine, guidelines pertaining to establishing a patient–provider relationship via telehealth, prescribing information, practice standards, consent requirements, out-of-state provider requirements, and certification requirements.
  - A patient's physical location is the site of service, and therefore, requires the nurse or provider to be licensed in that state. RNs and APRNs must verify the patient's location and the time services are rendered to ensure they are compliant.
  - All telehealth care provided by covered entities must comply with the Health Insurance Portability and Accountability Act rules.
- Neonatal telehealth care providers should strive for an equity-focused approach:
  - Understanding families' home environment and their life context is essential to providing high-quality telehealth care.
  - Providing culturally appropriate and language-concordant services is critical.
  - Telehealth care providers should be trained and competent in collaborating with medical interpreters.
- Programs, such as the Federal Communications Commission Wireless and Affordable Connectivity Program,[39] offer qualified Medicaid recipients and other eligible low-income families the opportunity to receive benefits, including a free smartphone with a discounted plan.
- Training and competencies must be delivered and evaluated in the health care setting for any provider engaging in telehealth with neonatal populations.

DISCLOSURE

The authors have no conflicts of interest to disclose.

REFERENCES

1. What is telehealth? US Department of Health and Human Services. Accessed August 16, 2023.
2. Lee EC, Grigorescu V, Enogieru I, et al. Updated national survey trends in telehealth utilization and modality (2021-2022), 2023, ASPE Assistant Secretary for Planning and Evaluation Office of Health Policy. https://aspe.hhs.gov/sites/default/files/documents/7d6b4989431f4c70144f209622975116/household-pulse-survey-telehealth-covid-ib.pdf.
3. 2021 Telehealth survey report. American Medical Association. Accessed August 23, 2023. https://www.ama-assn.org/system/files/telehealth-survey-report.pdf.

4. Altares Sarik D, Matsuda Y. Baby steps: improving the transition from hospital to home for neonatal patients and caregivers through a nurse-led telehealth program. In: Betz C, editor. *Worldwide successful pediatric nurse-led models of care.* Springer; 2022. p. 25–50. https://link.springer.com/book/10.1007/978-3-031-22152-1.

5. Sarik DA, Matsuda Y, Terrell EA, et al. A telehealth nursing intervention to improve the transition from the neonatal intensive care unit to home for infants & caregivers: preliminary evaluation. J Pediatr Nurs 2022;67:139–47.

6. Rasmussen MK, Clemensen J, Zachariassen G, et al. Cost analysis of neonatal tele-homecare for preterm infants compared to hospital-based care. J Telemed Telecare 2020;26(7–8):474–81.

7. Willard A, Brown E, Masten M, et al. Complex surgical infants benefit from post-discharge telemedicine visits. Adv Neonatal Care 2018;18(1):22–30.

8. Hoffman K, Olson C, Zenge J, et al. The use of telehealth to improve handoffs between neonatologists and primary care providers for medically complex infants, 2023, Telemedicine and e-Health. https://pubmed.ncbi.nlm.nih.gov/36877778/.

9. Jungbauer WN Jr, Gudipudi R, Brennan E, et al. The cost impact of telehealth interventions in pediatric surgical specialties: a systematic review. J Pediatr Surg 2022;58(8):1527–33.

10. Chuo J, Makkar A, Machut K, et al. Telemedicine across the continuum of neonatal-perinatal care. Semin Fetal Neonatal Med 2022;27(5):101398.

11. Sauers-Ford HS, Marcin JP, Underwood MA, et al. The use of telemedicine to address disparities in access to specialist care for neonates. Telemedicine and e-Health 2019;25(9):775–80.

12. Philip AG. The evolution of neonatology. Pediatr Res 2005;58(4):799–815.

13. Malloy MH, Wang LK. The limits of viability of extremely preterm infants. Baylor University Medical Center Proceedings 2022;35(5):731–5.

14. Kim Y, Ganduglia-Cazaban C, Chan W, et al. Trends in neonatal intensive care unit admissions by race/ethnicity in the United States, 2008–2018. Sci Rep 2021;11(1):23795.

15. Lor M, Crooks N, Tluczek A. A proposed model of person-family-and culture-centered nursing care. Nurs Outlook 2016;64(4):352–66.

16. Green J, Fowler C, Petty J, et al. The transition home of extremely premature babies: an integrative review. J Neonatal Nurs 2021;27(1):26–32.

17. Garber K, Chike-Harris K, Vetter MJ, et al. Telehealth policy and the advanced practice nurse. J Nurse Pract 2023;19(7):104655.

18. Avoiding the telehealth cliff ATA Action federal policy priorities in 2022. American Telehealth Association. Accessed August 16, 2023. https://www.americantelemed.org/wp-content/uploads/2022/11/ATA-Actions-2022-Legislative-Priorities-11.1.pdf.

19. Weigel G, Ramaswamy A, Sobel L, Salganicoff A, Cubanski J, Freed M. Opportunities and barriers for telemedicine in the U.S. during the COVID-19 emergency and beyond. KFF website. Accessed July 7, 2023. https://www.kff.org/womens-health-policy/issue-brief/opportunities-and-barriers-for-telemedicine-in-the-u-s-during-the-covid-19-emergency-and-beyond/.

20. Telehealth in the time of COVID-19. Center for Connected Health Policy. Accessed August 18, 2023. https://www.cchpca.org/covid-19-actions/.

21. Lin LA, Fernandez AC, Bonar EE. Telehealth for substance-using populations in the age of coronavirus disease 2019: recommendations to enhance adoption. JAMA Psychiatr 2020;77(12):1209–10.

22. Beaver NA, Lacktman NM, Ferrante TB, et al. DEA extends telemedicine flexibilities for prescribing of controlled medications. Health Care Law Today blog

2023;. https://www.foley.com/en/insights/publications/2023/05/dea-telemedicine-controlled-medications.

23. Garber KM, Chike-Harris KE. Nurse practitioners and virtual care: a 50-State review of APRN telehealth law and policy. Review. Telehealth and Medicine Today 2019;4:8.

24. Shaver J. The state of telehealth before and after the COVID-19 pandemic. Prim Care Clin Off Pract 2022;49(4):517–30.

25. State telehealth laws and Medicaid program policies. Center for Connected Health Policy. Accessed July 7, 2023. www.cchpca.org/2023/05/Spring2023_ExecutiveSummary.pdf.

26. Erikson C, Herring J, Park YH, et al. Association between state payment parity policies and telehealth usage at community health centers during COVID-19. J Am Med Inf Assoc 2022;29(10):1715–21.

27. Cross-state licensing. Center for Connected Health Policy. Accessed July 7, 2023. https://www.cchpca.org/topic/cross-state-licensing-covid-19/.

28. Benefits of the NLC. National Council of State Boards of Nursing. Accessed July 7, 2023. https://www.nursecompact.com/about.page.

29. APRN Compact benefits. National Council of State Boards of Nursing. Accessed July 7, 2023. https://www.aprncompact.com/about.page.

30. Position statement: telehealth. American Association of Nurse Practitioner. Accessed August 16, 2023. https://www.aanp.org/advocacy/advocacy-resource/position-statements/telehealth.

31. ANA core principles on connected health. American Nurses Association. Accessed August 23, 2023. https://www.nursingworld.org/~4a9307/globalassets/docs/ana/practice/ana-core-principles-on-connected-health.pdf.

32. ATA's federal telehealth legislative tracker. American Telemedicine Association. Accessed August 16, 2023. https://www.americantelemed.org/policies/atas-federal-telehealth-legislative-tracker/.

33. Health insurance portability and accountability act of 1996 (HIPAA). Centers for Disease Control and Prevention. Accessed July 7, 2023. https://www.cdc.gov/phlp/publications/topic/hipaa.html.

34. HIPAA rules for telehealth technology. US Department of Health and Human Services. Accessed August 16, 2023. https://telehealth.hhs.gov/providers/telehealth-policy/hipaa-for-telehealth-technology.

35. What is health equity? Centers for Disease Control and Prevention. Accessed July 7, 2023. https://www.cdc.gov/healthequity/whatis/index.html.

36. Social determinants of health. US Department of Health and Human Services. Accessed July 7, 2023. https://health.gov/healthypeople/priority-areas/social-determinants-health.

37. Mobile Fact Sheet. Pew Research Center. Accessed July 7, 2023. https://www.pewresearch.org/internet/fact-sheet/mobile/.

38. Vogels EA. Digital divide persists as Americans with lower income make gains in tech adoption. Pew Research Center. https://www.pewresearch.org/short-reads/2021/06/22/digital-divide-persists-even-as-americans-with-lower-incomes-make-gains-in-tech-adoption. Accessed August 16, 2023.

39. Affordable connectivity program. Federal Communications Commission. https://www.fcc.gov/acp. Accessed August 16, 2023.

40. Huvila I. Information services and digital literacy. *Information Services and digital literacy in Search of the Boundaries of knowing*, 2012, Elsevier, 25–34, Chandos Information Professional Series. https://www.sciencedirect.com/book/9781843346838/information-services-and-digital-literacy.

41. Samuels-Kalow ME, Chary AN, Ciccolo G, et al. Barriers and facilitators to pediatric telehealth use in English-and Spanish-speaking families: a qualitative study. J Telemed Telecare 2022. 1357633X211070725.

42. National CLAS standards. US Department of Health and Human Services. https://thinkculturalhealth.hhs.gov/clas. Accessed August 16, 2023.

43. Cultural competence in health and human services. Centers for Disease Control and Prevention. https://npin.cdc.gov/pages/cultural-competence. Accessed July 7, 2023.

44. Hook JN, Davis DE, Owen J, et al. Cultural humility: measuring openness to culturally diverse clients. J Counsel Psychol 2013;60(3):353.

45. Tervalon M, Murray-Garcia J. Cultural humility versus cultural competence: a critical distinction in defining physician training outcomes in multicultural education. J Health Care Poor Underserved 1998;9(2):117–25.

46. Williams R. Cultural safety—what does it mean for our work practice? Aust N Z J Publ Health 1999;23(2):213–4.

47. Koukourikos K, Tsaloglidou A, Kourkouta L, et al. Simulation in clinical nursing education. Acta Inf Med 2021;29(1):15.

48. Matsuda Y, Valdes B, Salani DA, et al. Baby Steps Program: telehealth nursing simulation for undergraduate public health nursing students. Clinical simulation in nursing 2022;65:35–44.

49. Watkins S, Neubrander J. Primary-care registered nurse telehealth policy implications. J Telemed Telecare 2022;28(3):203–6.

50. Creating a framework to support measure development for telehealth. National Quality Forum. https://www.qualityforum.org/Publications/2017/08/Creating_a_Framework_to_Support_Measure_Development_for_Telehealth.aspx. Accessed August 16, 2023.

51. Monitoring and evaluating digital health interventions: a practical guide to conducting research and assessment. World Health Organization. https://apps.who.int/iris/bitstream/handle/10665/252183/9789241511766-eng.pdf?sequence=1&isAllowed=y.

52. Totten A, Womack DM, Eden KB, McDonagh M, Griffin J, Hersh W. Telehealth: mapping the evidence for patient outcomes from systematic reviews. Agency for Healthcare Research and Quality. Available at: https://effectivehealthcare.ahrq.gov/sites/default/files/pdf/telehealth_technical-brief.pdf. Accessed July 7, 2023.

53. Chuo J, Macy ML, Lorch SA. Strategies for evaluating telehealth. Pediatrics 2020;146(5):e20201781.

Neonatal Nursing Care from a Global Perspective

Carole Kenner, PhD, RN, ANEF, IDFCOINN[a,b,*],
Marina Boykova, PhD, RN, PNAP[a,c]

KEYWORDS

- Neonatal nursing • Global • Workforce • Neonatal nursing education

KEY POINTS

- Neonatal mortality has stagnated and, in some instances, worsened.
- On a global level, neonatal nursing is not recognized as a special field of nursing.
- Strengthening the neonatal nursing workforce is essential to changing neonatal/family outcomes.

INTRODUCTION

In May 2023, the World Health Organization (WHO) launched the second edition of the *"Born Too Soon: Decade of Action on Preterm Birth"* opening with the frightening statement that globally, "every 2 seconds a baby is born prematurely."[1(p13)] This statistic coupled with the fact that "preterm births account for the majority of under 5 years of age deaths."[1(p13)] Moreover, complications of preterm birth account for 0.9 million neonatal deaths annually.[1] Unfortunately, in the last few years, maternal and neonatal mortality rates have stagnated or only minimally decreased.[1] For example, in 2020 in Zimbabwe neonatal mortality rate (NMR) was 25.55 per 1000 live births; it only decreased to 24.99 per 1000 live births in 2021.[2] In 2020 in Nigeria, the NMR was 35.48, and in 2021, it was 34.92 per 1000 live births.[2] Although both countries demonstrated a decline in neonatal mortality,[2] it was a negligible change. In the United States, the same trend is noted with 3.38 in 2020 as compared with 3.27 deaths per 1000 live births in 2021.[2] None of these figures is close to the Sustainable Development Goal #3.2 target of 12 deaths per 1000 live births.[1]

Since the first edition of the "Born Too Soon" report came out in 2012, slow progress has been made.[3] Why? It is suggested that there are 4 factors affecting global mortality in mothers and infants (4 Cs): conflicts, climate change, coronavirus disease 2019

---

[a] Council of International Neonatal Nurses, Inc. (COINN); [b] School of Nursing & Health Sciences, The College of New Jersey; [c] School of Nursing and Health Sciences, Holy Family University, 9801 Frankford Avenue, Philadelphia, PA 19114, USA
* Corresponding author. The College of New Jersey, 2000 Pennington Road, Ewing, NJ 08628.
E-mail addresses: kennerc@tcnj.edu; ceo@coinnurses.org

Crit Care Nurs Clin N Am 36 (2024) 147–156
https://doi.org/10.1016/j.cnc.2023.08.005
0899-5885/24/© 2023 Elsevier Inc. All rights reserved.

(COVID-19), and the cost-of-living crisis.[1] No doubt, these factors negatively influence maternal and newborn health; however, in our opinion, quality nursing care for neonates and their mothers is the key factor in decreasing deaths in these vulnerable populations. However, only well-educated and well-trained nurses can provide a high-quality care. High mortality rates translate to a need for specialized training and education in the nursing workforce that cares for small and sick newborns. At present, neonatal nursing is at the forefront of global policymaking and workforce discussions. Hopefully, investments by governments in neonatal nursing education/training will lead to better health outcomes, as demonstrated in high-income countries.[4] This article will address neonatal nursing specialization/education/workforce issues that are affecting neonatal mortality and neonatal nursing care globally; the role professional associations play in improving neonatal nursing education, and practice is discussed.

NEONATAL NURSING ORGANIZATIONS AND THEIR ROLES: SOME EXAMPLES

Neonatal nursing as a specialization has been around for decades but, not in every country. In the United Kingdom (UK), the United States (US), Canada, Australia, and New Zealand, neonatal nurses formed early neonatal nursing associations. The Neonatal Nurses Association (NNA) was established in the UK in 1977 in response to high perinatal mortality.[5] In the US, the National Association of Neonatal Nurses (NANN) was established in 1984[6] followed by the Australian College of Neonatal Nurses (ACNN)[7] in 1992 and New Zealand Neonatal Nurses in 1995 (later named Neonatal Nurses College of Aotearoa as a part of New Zealand Nurses Organization) (O'Donoghue D. Personal communication. About Neonatal Nurses College Aotearoa. July 12, 2023).[8] In the US, the Academy of Neonatal Nursing was formed in 2001.[9] The Canadian Association of Neonatal Nurses (CANN) was also launched in 2006,[10] and the Neonatal Nurses Association of Southern Africa (NNASA) was formed in 2007.[11]

The professional associations set standards for neonatal nursing education and practice. They offer definitions of a neonatal nurse and advanced practice nurse (eg, neonatal nurse practitioner in the US). Working in tandem with medical and midwifery colleagues, competencies are identified that support neonatal education/ orientation/training. These organizations also develop clinical performance indicators that translate into more standardized neonatal nursing practice. Yet, in many countries, especially in low-resourced ones, the neonatal nursing specialty is not recognized. No consistency exists for what a neonatal nurse can do while providing care for a newborn. Responsibilities, tasks, and levels of autonomy widely vary. There is often no scope of practice set in a country, but rather, an institution determines the nurse's role. This is why an international organization was needed.

In 2005, the Council of International Neonatal Nurses, Inc (COINN)[12] was formed to address the need for neonatal nursing to be recognized as a specialization, to bring nursing's voice to the policy tables, and to increase the visibility of the role neonatal nurses play in decreasing infant mortality and improving health outcomes. NANN, NNA, ACNN, NNASA, and CANN were the founding organizations for COINN. At present, there are 16 national organizations involved in COINN, and collectively, more than 6000 nurses are represented by this council. COINN unites nurses who provide care to newborns and their families all over the globe. COINN helps these nurses organize neonatal nursing organizations, organize conferences, develop international and country-specific competencies, and provides educational opportunities. For instance, COINN was asked by neonatologists and nurses from India to help launch an organization to address neonatal mortality and neonatal nursing staffing challenges. The India Neonatal Nurses Association was formed in 2007. In 2018, the Rwanda

Association of Neonatal Nurses launched as well followed in 2019 by the Kenya Neonatal Nurses Association. Zambia was about to launch its organization in 2020 when the COVID-19 pandemic hit.

ADDRESSING NEONATAL AND MATERNAL HEALTH OUTCOMES

Neonatal and maternal mortality rates are key indicators of a country's well-being and level of development. Efforts to address the needs of these vulnerable populations have been made for a long time. For instance, in 1976, the March of Dimes (MOD, USA-based organization) published *"Toward Improving the Outcome of Pregnancy"*[13] that outlined the need for more consistent training of the workforce in maternal child health. Regionalization models of care and training were created where interprofessional teams would come to a tertiary center to learn new skills and see new advanced care techniques. The American Academy of Pediatrics (AAP) Committee on Fetus and Newborn worked with the American College of Obstetricians and Gynecologists to publish *"Guidelines for Perinatal Care"* (now in its eighth edition)[14]–and one nurse was included as a member of this committee by the mid-1990s. The nurse brought the perspective of neonatal *nursing* care, conveying an additional dimension to the development of the guidelines. This document describes the stabilization of the newborn, staffing, transport, infection control, and management of the high-risk infant.[14]

Every country has its own standards and protocols of care. Some countries provide better health care than others. The launch of the Lancet series on Neonatal Survival occurred in 2005 and brought attention to inappropriately high NMRs. It catalyzed action to develop targets to improve neonatal outcomes and under-5 years of age mortality rates.[15] Globally, most neonatal deaths occurred in Sub-Saharan Africa and were due to infection and asphyxia-preventable causes.[16] This study raised awareness that premature births were a significant public health problem influencing society's welfare. The publications were aligned with the United Nations (UN) Millennium Development Goals (MDGs) that were launched in 2000 to outline a blueprint for countries to improve health. Specifically, MDG #4 addressed the reduction of child mortality.[17] By 2015, the under-5 years of age mortality rate was reduced from 90 to 43 deaths per 1000 live births.[17] Although the progress in decreasing child mortality was demonstrated, it was not enough as the question arose—was this decrease sustainable? In 2016, the UN launched the 17 Sustainable Development Goals (SDGs) with goal #3 emphasizing Good Health and Well-Being.[18] By 2020, the global mortality rate for children aged younger than 5 years dropped by 14% from the 2015 rate.[18]

Through the SDGs, targets are set to address key areas that require action by the countries with the highest neonatal and child mortality under 5 years of age. According to SDG, the specific targets for neonatal mortality are set at 12 per 1000 live births and under-5 years of age mortality at 25 per 1000 live births.[18] Strengthening the nursing workforce through financial support, recruitment, training/education, and retention is a key recommendation.[18] The "how" to achieve targets was discussed in the WHO's 2014 work *"Every Newborn Action Plan"* (ENAP) that outlined strategic actions for "ending preventable newborn mortality and stillbirth and contributing to reducing maternal mortality and morbidity."[19] The second part of this work, *"Ending Preventable Maternal Mortality"* (EPMM) aims at improving maternal health through accessible and high-quality care and links with the ENAP objectives.[20]

ENAP/EPMM calls for alliances across civil society, professional organizations, and governmental and nongovernmental agencies. Many alliances were created, and one example of a broad collaboration is the Newborn Essential Solutions and

Technologies (NEST 360), which represents "an international alliance united to end preventable newborn deaths in African hospitals."[21] Partners include many global foundations, health-care organizations, and nongovernmental, governmental, and health professional groups. The study focuses on strengthening the health-care delivery system, making health care accessible to mothers and newborns, and training/educating a cadre of health professionals. Until recently, midwives and physicians were the focus of this training in most cases. However, things changed in 2020 when neonatal nurses received long-awaited attention.

In 2020, the WHO launched a *"Human Resources Strategies Roadmap" (HRH)*, and, for the first time, neonatal nursing was included as a key part of the health-care workforce.[22] This roadmap called for strengthening the cadre of existing nurses and training new cadres of nurses who were well trained and educated to take care of small and sick newborns.[22] This recognition—that nurses are the frontline workers that are most involved with the newborn and family and that nurses must be adequately trained—brought new opportunities.

The WHO's *"Recommendations for Care of the Preterm or Low-Birth-Weight Infant,"* released on World Prematurity Day in November 2022, are changing practice.[23] These updated evidence-based recommendations included neonatal nurses and parents as part of the development team. This report states that "approximately 45% of all children under the age of five who die are newborns, and 60% to 80% of those newborns who die are premature and/or small for gestational age." (24, p.vii) The authors proposed 25 recommendations and one good-practice statement.[23] New recommendations include the call for immediate KMC, the use of probiotics for human-milk-fed very preterm infants, the application of emollients, and specific uses of CPAP and caffeine. A new section addresses family involvement, support, home visits, and parental leave and entitlements.[23] The implementation of these recommendations will change practice and neonatal/family outcomes. However, these changes will only be successful with a knowledgeable, well-trained health-care workforce—including nurses.

Role of Council of International Neonatal Nurses, Inc

COINN, as the only voice for global neonatal nurses, worked on each of global initiatives mentioned above, first by endorsing reports and then by attending United Nations (UN) meetings where the first *"Born Too Soon"* report was launched in 2012.[3] COINN participated in several side meetings at the UN where ENAP targets were endorsed. COINN joined the International Council of Nurses as an associate member and became a member of the WHO Partnership for Maternal, Newborn, Child, and Adolescent Health Healthcare Professional Associations constituency. As of now, CONN continues to contribute to the writing of policies and reports.

One of the major parts of COINN's study is neonatal nursing workforce issues. In 2018, COINN conducted a survey in Rwanda to determine neonatal nursing practices in relationship to orientation, education, and skill levels as well as available equipment to provide neonatal care.[24] Ninety-nine midwives, nurse-midwives, and nurses from all 47 neonatal care units in Rwanda participated.[24] The results showed a lack of consistent orientation and training for those providing care, comfort with basic caregiving skills but not advanced ones, and a lack of equipment.[24] Some participants stated that the doctors who backed them up in the neonatal care units also lacked training in small and sick newborns and were not available all 24 hours.[24] The nurses/midwives were the only frontline workers in many instances. Based on these findings and the data from focus groups of Rwandan nurses at an in-country 2019 COINN conference, COINN developed a competency-based curriculum for preservice (training before earning a college degree) and in-service training.[25] This framework for this curriculum draws from competencies and curricular models found in the US, UK, Australia, New Zealand, and the International Confederation of Midwives. COINN also began to work with universities that requested assistance in developing bachelor's and master's levels neonatal nursing education models. COINN developed competencies to guide educational content and practice. A clinical skills checklist accompanied these competencies to measure clinical performance.[26] Consistent curricular content that reflects the expected competencies needed for each of the 3 levels of WHO care is essential if nurses are to be better prepared to take care of small and sick newborns.[22]

COINN has partnered with organizations such as Project Hope, USAID, WHO, Save The Children, and others to bring expertise in neonatal care and education. In the last few years, trainings were held in Nigeria (virtually), Ghana (virtually and on the ground), Zambia (virtually and on the ground), and Rwanda (on the ground), and students from many other African countries have joined the online training community. COINN has launched a Community of Neonatal Nursing Practice (CoNP) (https://www.conp communityofpractice.org) to provide curricular outlines, resources from many organizations, best practices/guidelines for care, and a place to discuss challenges and opportunities. This CoNP links to other communities of practice, such as the Care of the Small and Sick Newborn Community of Practice, to amplify the resources available at this site. The WHO *Essential Newborn Care*[27] is another resource for training across disciplines, and community health works that are on the CoNP. These communities of practice are rich with evidence-based guidelines, standards, and skill-based resources. Sharing through these communities will help change practice.

DISCUSSION

Partnerships are very important for improving patient outcomes. By joining forces with other organizations, including interprofessional ones, partnerships amplify the efforts of an individual organization to improve the health of global society members. From 1969 through the 1980s, early nursing specialty organizations were formed, and new partnerships for improving given care occurred. For example, in the US, the Nurses Association of the American College of Obstetricians and Gynecologists (now the Association for Women's Health, Obstetrics, and Neonatal Nurses) and the NANN brought the maternal child and neonatal nurses together to share best practices and learn from each other. These US organizations started to develop standards for neonatal nursing care, education, and training/orientation and raised the visibility of the role neonatal nurses play in health outcomes for the baby and family.

There are a few similar nursing organizations in low-resourced countries—countries where the NMRs are unacceptably high. At present, the situation in many low-resourced countries is very similar to what it was like in the US in the 1970s and 1980s when nurses were assigned to work the neonatal units with little orientation and no specific neonatal training, when each institution developed the orientations, there was lack of consistency in these programs. In addition to the lack of good education and training in countries with high NMR, there are often problems with staffing, nurse–patient ratios, and equipment. Imam and colleagues[28] conducted a systematic review that examined missed care and the areas of care most likely to be missed in acute care settings. They found that nurses prioritized task-oriented care over the soft skills of communication and compassion, leading to quality care and patient safety issues.[28] The reason given was staffing—not enough staff.[28] The researchers suggested that improved staffing and task shifting of those activities that could be done by others might help improve the situation.[28] Dr. Imam presented his study (conducted in the Kenyan newborn units) at the May 2023 ALIGNMNH conference in Cape Town, South Africa.[29] He reported that for the 8 hospitals participating in the study, the staffing nurse/infant ratios were 1:14 for the day shift and 1:24 for the night shift.[29] The mean nursing hours per patient ranged from 20.4 to 64.4 minutes.[29] Nurses spent a lot of time on IV medications and little time on other activities, leading to potential safety issues and lower quality of care.[29] Unfortunately, Such a practice environment is not unusual for low-resourced countries. If we want to decrease global NMRs, the staffing ratios should be smaller (aka safer) than what was reported in this study.

So, what can be done to help nurses to provide the best possible care to help babies survive and thrive? We believe that 3 things can do it: education, empowerment, and professional organizations.

Today, high-resourced countries have educational pathways to advanced practice nursing—at a master's or doctoral level. Neonatal nurses earn science-based degrees such as the Doctor of Philosophy (PhD) in nursing. Orientation programs exist, although some of these have been abbreviated due to the pandemic and the increasing shortage of nurses (nationally and globally). No doubt, nurses who provide care to small and sick newborns in low-resourced settings all need to know the basics—how to stabilize a newborn, provide resuscitation, and promote and teach families how to do Kangaroo Mother Care (KMC). However, they also need advanced knowledge of fetal development, neonatal physiology, pathophysiology, pharmacology, and health assessment. If we are to tackle global neonatal deaths, the basic knowledge of newborn care is not enough—nurses need (and want!) more knowledge and information on how to help a sick or small baby. For example, according to COINN's survey in Rwanda, nurses reported that they want to learn more about continuous positive pressure ventilation, skillfully perform resuscitation and stabilization, and learn about surgical/genetic malformations and infections. It is worth noting that many African countries are using the AAP Helping Babies Breathe[30] as well as the Neonatal Resuscitation Program[31] and the S.T.A.B.L.E. program, which was developed by a nurse.[32] WHO also developed the *Essential Newborn Care*[30] that covers immediate care—KMC, breastfeeding, delayed cord clamping, drying, assessment of breathing, thermoregulation, resuscitation, nurturing care, infection prevention, danger signs, and referrals when needed.[30] All these programs effectively reduce neonatal mortality when providers are adequately trained; however, nurses (especially with limited access to neonatal care training, education, and informational resources) want to know more—in essence, everything well beyond the basics. WHO is beginning to move beyond the basics to modular and more advanced courses that are needed so much.

Organizing the neonatal nursing workforce and empowerment are vitally important for improving neonatal outcomes. Care improves when nursing concerns about their training needs and how care is delivered are heard and addressed by policymakers and administrators. Bringing nurses and nurse champions together with neonatologists, pediatricians, nursing councils, and ministries of health to practical issues/policy discussion tables will result in change at the grassroots/higher levels. The exchange of knowledge and best practices is a must in this contemporary world that is globally connected and interwoven in any aspect of human lives. Reviewing some of the history of neonatal care and the impact that interprofessional policymakers have had on outcomes is important. Developing leadership and mentorship nursing programs, and international networking builds confidence and empowers nurses to achieve their full potential. Empowered nurses change practice. International organizations such as COINN help local organizations to be involved at the global level and address their national needs appropriately. As we said above, COINN has supported the launch of associations in India, South Africa, Rwanda, and Kenya—and other Sub-Saharan African countries are willing to establish their own neonatal nursing organizations. The efforts are aimed at the countries with the biggest needs and those that have the worst NMRs. Many groups are operationalizing the *WHO HRH Roadmap*,[22] helping achieve the targets and replicating educational programs that high-resourced countries have demonstrated to improve health outcomes. No doubt, technological advances, and breakthroughs in care and treatments (such as surfactant, nitric oxide, high-tech equipment, and effective medications/vaccines against infections), all improve infant outcomes but still, the key role of a well-educated and competent neonatal nurse cannot be overlooked or overemphasized. In the US, nurses continue to contribute to country-level guidelines such as *"Guidelines for Perinatal Care,"* yet there is still only one nurse on this committee[14] and globally nurses are often still absent from national guidelines' development in many countries, high-resourced or low-resourced. This situation must be changed if we want to decrease global NMRs. COINN continues working with an international cadre of nurse/physician/midwife educators to offer advanced training/education, partnering with universities to develop bachelor's and master's-level programs. COINN also partners with many programs that are already available; however, we need to do more for newborn infants over the globe.

One more important thing that cannot be missed is the presence of parents of newborn infants. Parents must be included in practice/policy discussions because they know the newborn unit/neonatal intensive care unit (NICU) practices from upside down, and they have invaluable experiences to share with health-care professionals that would benefit babies and health-care systems. Parent groups exist in many countries and should be involved to bring their perspective to neonatal care. However, parents are often forgotten despite the fact that they are key decision-makers and key caregivers for an infant's health and life. There are very strong and powerful parental organizations in the Western world but not in all countries. Examples of parent support groups include Preemie Parent Alliance, Preemie World, Alliance for Black NICU Families in the US, Miracle Babies in Australia, Preemie Connect in South Africa, and Little Big Souls in Africa. Another very strong parental organization is the European Foundation for the Care of Newborn Infants, which was involved in working with WHO, COINN, and many other international organizations to develop the new WHO Recommendations Care of the Preterm or Low-Birthweight Infants.[23] We believe that having strong parental organizations in countries with high NMRs would benefit practice and policy changes to decrease neonatal deaths. At the ALIGNNMNH conference, where the *"Born Too Soon"*[1] latest edition was launched (Collective action for maternal newborn health https://www.alignmnh.org/), the organizers presented parental stories that moved many health-care professionals. At the beginning of the conference, one of the keynote speakers was a mother with a very inspiring name, Treasure, talking about her experience of having a preterm baby. We need to use these parent experiences for infant and family outcomes.

SUMMARY

At present, neonatal nursing is at the forefront of all policy discussions that focus on neonatal or under 5 years of age mortality because recognition is growing about the role these nurses play in neonatal outcomes. Nursing is included to bring real-world experience to often theoretic dialogs. Standards are being developed with in-country representatives to reflect cultural values, beliefs, and availability of equipment and support services. Neonatal nursing experts from around the world are mentoring faculty who are responsible for teaching small and sick newborn content; experts are teaching courses to students globally—some virtually through the pandemic and beyond followed, when possible, in-country in the neonatal units. Experts come into the country to provide "train-the-trainer" sessions so they can take over the in-country training. Other experts act as preceptors supervising the students and teaching the doctors what fully trained nurses can do. For neonatal nursing, our time has come to be recognized as an essential member of the small and sick newborn team who must be adequately prepared to deliver high-quality care. Specialty education and consistent, competency-based training are being made available in some countries in Africa but this opportunity needs to spread. Neonatal mortality can only change if neonatal nurses are trained/educated on the care delivery of small and sick newborns. In the last few years, less progress has been made to reduce these deaths. Nurses and sometimes doctors or midwives who take care of the most vulnerable newborns have no specific training or education on the physiologic differences, pathologic conditions, or medications and treatments. At this moment in time, leaders of civil society, policymakers, professional organizations, universities, ministries of health, and nursing councils are working together for a call to action to have a better-prepared workforce. Only when this becomes a reality will neonatal mortality globally decrease and preventable death averted. The ALIGNNMNH offered the mantra, "This is not a moment in time, but a movement!" For neonatal nurses, we are a critical part of that movement.

CLINICS CARE POINTS

- A better-prepared workforce equates to better health outcomes and higher-quality care.
- Care practices are difficult to shift even with mounting evidence to the contrary.
- Neonatal care will not change if the education/training of the workforce is not scaled up.

DISCLOSURE

Nothing to disclose.

REFERENCES

1. World Health Organization (WHO). Born too soon: Decade of action on preterm birth. 2023. https://www.who.int/publications/i/item/9789240073890. Accessed July 27, 2023.
2. UNICEF. UNICEF Data warehouse. 2023. https://data.unicef.org/resources/data_explorer/unicef_f/?ag=UNICEF&df=GLOBAL_DATAFLOW&ver=1.0&dq=ZWE.CME_MRM0.&startPeriod=1970&endPeriod=2023. Accessed July 27, 2023.
3. World Health Organization. Born too soon: the global action report on preterm birth. World Health Organization; 2021. https://apps.who.int/iris/handle/10665/44864. Accessed July 28, 2023.
4. Lasater KB, Sloane DM, McHugh MD, et al. Changes in proportion of bachelor's nurses associated with improvements in patient outcomes. Res Nurs Health 2021;44(5):787–95.
5. Neonatal Nurses Association. About the NNA, 2023; http://www.nna.org.uk/about.html. Accessed July 27, 2023.

6. National Association of Neonatal Nurses (NANN). History. 2023: https://nann.org/about/history. Accessed July 27, 2023.
7. Australian College of Neonatal Nurses (ACNN). About. 2023; https://www.acnn.org.au/about/acnn/. Accessed July 27, 2023.
8. Neonatal Nurses College of Aotearoa. In this area. 2023; https://nzno.org.nz/groups/colleges_sections/colleges/neonatal_nurses_college. Accessed July 27, 2023.
9. Academy of neonatal nursing. 2023; https://www.academyonline.org/. Accessed July 28, 2023.
10. Canadian Association of Neonatal Nurses. (CANN). About CANN. https://neonatalcann.ca/about-us. Accessed July 27, 2023.
11. Healthy Newborn Network. Neonatal nurses association of southern Africa. https://www.healthynewbornnetwork.org/partner/neonatal-nurses-association-southern-africa/. Accessed July 27, 2023.
12. Council of International Neonatal Nurses. (COINN). About COINN, 2023: https://www.coinnurses.org/about-us. Accessed July 28, 2023.
13. March of Dimes (MOD). Toward improving the outcome of pregnancy. White Plains, NY: MOD; 1976.
14. American Academy of Pediatrics (AAP). Committee on Fetus and newborn and American college of Obstetrics & gynecology (ACOG) committee on obstetric practice. In: Kilpatrick SJ, Papile L-A, Macones GA, et al, editors. guidelines for perinatal care. 8th edition. elk gorve village, IL: American Academy of Pediatrics and American college of Obstetricians and Gynecologists; 2017.
15. Marines J, Paul VK, Bhutta ZA, et al. Lancet neonatal survival steering team. Neonatal survival: a call for action. Lancet 2005;365(9465):1189–97.
16. Lawn JE, Cousens S, Zupan J, et al. Lancet neonatal survival steering team. 4 million neonatal deaths: when? Where? Why. Lancet 2005;365(9462):891–900. PMID: 15752534.
17. United Nations. (UN). We can end poverty: Millennium development goals and beyond 2015; https://www.un.org/millenniumgoals/. Accessed June 12, 2023.
18. United Nations (UN). Sustainable development goals. 2015; https://www.un.org/sustainabledevelopment/health/. Accessed June 12, 2023.
19. World Health Organization (WHO). Every newborn action plan. 2014: https://www.who.int/initiatives/every-newborn-action-plan. Accessed June 12, 2023.
20. World Health Organization (WHO). Ending preventable maternal mortality (EPMM). 2015; https://www.who.int/initiatives/ending-preventable-maternal-mortality. Accessed June 12, 2023.
21. Unicef. NEST360. 2023; https://nest360.org/. Accessed June 12, 2023.
22. World Health Organization (WHO). Human resource strategies to improve newborn care in health facilities in low- and middle-income countries. Geneva: World Health Organization; 2020. License CC BY-NC-SA=2.0 IGO. https://www.who.int/news/item/17-11-2020. Accessed June 12, 2023.
23. World Health Organization (WHO). WHO recommendations for care of the preterm or low- birth-weight infant. Geneva: World Health Organization; 2022. License: CC BY-NC-SA 3.0 IGO. https://www.who.int/publications/i/item/9789240058262. Accessed July 28, 2023.
24. Prullage GS, Kenner C, Uwingabire F, et al. Survey of neonatal nursing: staffing, education, and equipment availability in Rwanda. J Neonatal Nurs 2018;28(3):192–9.
25. Jones T. International neonatal nursing competency framework. J Neonatal Nurs 2019;24(50):258–64.

26. Prullage GS, Walker K, Kenner C, et al. Integrating a skills checklist into the CO-INN neonatal nurse competencies. J Neonatal Nurs 2022;28(3):200–2.

27. World Health Organization (WHO). Essential newborn care. 2023: https://www.who.int/teams/maternal-newborn-child-adolescent-health-and-ageing/newborn-health/essential-newborn-care. Accessed July 28, 2023.

28. Imam A, Obiesie S, Gathara D, et al. Missed nursing care in acute care hospital settings in low-income and middle-income countries: a systematic review. Hum Resource Health 2023;21(19). Accessed July 28, 2023.

29. Imam A. Missed nursing care and informal task shifting within Kenyan newborn units: relationship with nurse staffing and care quality. Cape Town, South Africa: ALIGNNMNH; 2023.

30. American Academy of Pediatrics (AAP). Helping babies breathe. 2023: https://www.aap.org/en/aap-global/helping-babies-survive/our-programs/helping-babies breathe/. Accessed July 28, 2023.

31. American Academy of Pediatrics (AAP). Neonatal resuscitation program (NRP). 2023; https://aap.org/en/learning/neonatal-resuscitation-program/. Accessed July 28, 2023.

32. Karlsen KA. The S.T.A.B.L.E. Program. Park City, Utah: S.T.A.B.L.E; 2023. https://stableprogram.org/. Accessed June 15, 2023.

Moving?

Make sure your subscription moves with you!

To notify us of your new address, find your **Clinics Account Number** (located on your mailing label above your name), and contact customer service at:

Email: journalscustomerservice-usa@elsevier.com

800-654-2452 (subscribers in the U.S. & Canada)
314-447-8871 (subscribers outside of the U.S. & Canada)

Fax number: 314-447-8029

Elsevier Health Sciences Division
Subscription Customer Service
3251 Riverport Lane
Maryland Heights, MO 63043

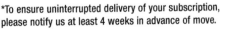
*To ensure uninterrupted delivery of your subscription, please notify us at least 4 weeks in advance of move.

Printed and bound by CPI Group (UK) Ltd, Croydon, CR0 4YY

03/10/2024

01040473-0015